ITALIAN COOKING

50 Classic Italian Delicious and Easy to Prepare Recipes to Stay Fit and Live Healthy

John P. Leone

PUBLISHED BY: Green Book Publishing LTD

24 Tax Suite 137 B Westlink House 981 Great West Road Brentford, United Kingdom, TW8 9DN

First Print 2021

Copyright 2021 © John P. Leone

Green Book Publishing ®

All rights reserved. No part of this guide may be reproduced in any form without permission in writing from the publisher except in the case of brief quotations embodied in critical articles or reviews.

Legal & Disclaimer

The information contained in this book and its contents is not designed to replace or take the place of any form of medical or professional advice; and is not meant to replace the need for independent medical, financial, legal or other professional advice or services, as may be required. The content and information in this book has been provided for educational and entertainment purposes only.

The content and information contained in this book has been compiled from sources deemed reliable, and it is accurate to the best of the Author's knowledge, information and belief. However, the Author cannot guarantee its accuracy and validity and cannot be held liable for any errors and/or omissions. Further, changes are periodically made to this book as and when needed. Where appropriate and/or necessary, you must consult a professional (including but not limited to your doctor, attorney, financial advisor or such other professional advisor) before using any of the suggested remedies, techniques, or information in this book.

Upon using the contents and information contained in this book, you agree to hold harmless the Author from and against any damages, costs, and expenses, including any legal fees potentially resulting from the application of any of the information provided by this book. This disclaimer applies to any loss, damages or injury caused by the use and application, whether directly or indirectly, of any advice or information presented, whether for breach of contract, tort, negligence, personal injury, criminal intent, or under any other cause of action.

You agree to accept all risks of using the information presented inside this book.

You agree that by continuing to read this book, where appropriate and/or necessary, you shall consult a professional (including but not limited to your doctor, attorney, or financial advisor or such other advisor as needed) before using any of the suggested remedies, techniques, or information in this book.

Table of Contents

Appetizers 9
   Shrimp Appetizer 9
   Mussels Appetizer 11
   Mushroom Appetizer 13
   Anchovies with Lemon 15
   Sicilian Arancini 17
   Cheese Puffs 19
   Ascolana Olives 21
   Broccoli Batter 23
   Baked Ham Croquettes 25
   Cheese Patties 27

Main Courses 29
   Cannelloni with Spinach 29
   Pumpkin Tortelli 32
   Timbale of Fusilli 34
   Orecchiette with Cauliflower 36
   Macaroni with Artichokes 38
   Farfalle with Mushroom Sauce 40
   Fettuccine with Salmon 42
   Pasta with Sardines 44
   Rice with Peas and Cheese 46
   Mushroom Risotto 48
   Baked Lamb 50

Ossibuchi with Mushrooms 52

Turkey with Potatoes 54

Beef with Mushrooms 56

Pork with Corn 58

Cod with Lemon 60

Lobster with Spices 62

Trout and Nuts 64

Sea Bream with Baked Potatoes 66

Perch with Cherry Tomatoes and Basil 68

Side Dishes 70

Parmigiana Asparagus 70

Piemontese Polenta 72

Carrot Puree 74

Mexican Beans 76

Stuffed Champignons 78

Baked Zucchini 80

Sautéed Mushrooms 82

Corn Salad 84

Breaded Artichokes 86

Sauteed Broccoli 88

Sweet and Treats 90

Italian Babà 90

Cinnamon Cookies 92

Eggnog 94

Hazelnut Ice Cream 95

Profiteroles 97
Sweet Salami.. 100
Lemon Sorbet 102
Cannoncini with Cream 104
Coffee Chocolates.. 106
Blueberry Jam 108

Welcome to this amazing guide! If you decided to buy this book it means you have a passion for cooking and food! So, let me compliment you!

Being curious and wanting to learn new things is synonymous with intelligence, and this is certainly no exception for cooking. In this book I deal with very simple, but at the same time delicious recipes; these are quick but very engaging recipes. I assure you that you will amaze the guests you invite for lunch or dinner to let them taste your delicacies. But, more importantly, you will amaze yourself!

You will expand your culinary horizons; you will learn new dishes to prepare and above all you will be satisfied with what you will be able to do!

So, after this short introduction, let's dive right into the practice!

Enjoy!

Appetizers

Shrimp Appetizer

Ingredients: 6 servings

- Shrimp, 500 gr.
- 1 lemon
- Parsley, to taste
- Olive oil, to taste
- Salt and pepper, to taste

Direction:

1) Wash the shrimp. Put them on the fire in lightly salted cold water. Boil them for two or three minutes and then drain them.

2) Shell the shrimp. Put them on the serving dish. Season them still hot with lemon, parsley, olive oil and pepper. Serve and enjoy your meal!

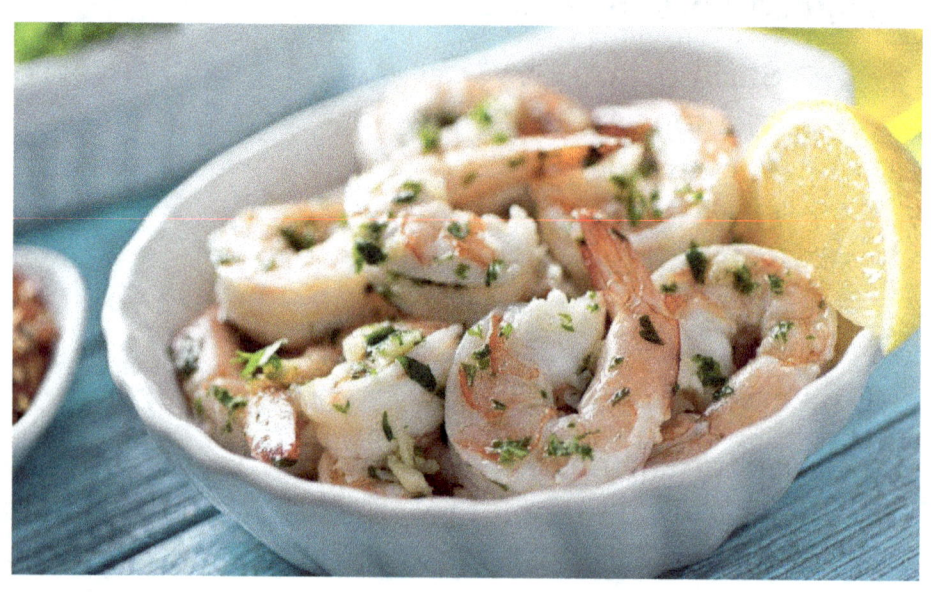

Mussels Appetizer

Ingredients: 2 servings

- Mussels, 1 kg
- Squid, 150 gr.
- 1 red pepper
- Lemon, ½
- Salt and Pepper, to taste
- Green and black olives, 50 gr.
- Extra virgin olive oil, to taste
- Capers, 25 gr.

Directions:

1) Put the mussels to open in a pan on the fire. Cook the squid. Slice into julienne strips. Mix the squid fillets with the mussels.

2) Combine julienne sliced capers and peppers. Season with salt, pepper, a drizzle of extra virgin olive oil and lemon juice. Enjoy your meal!

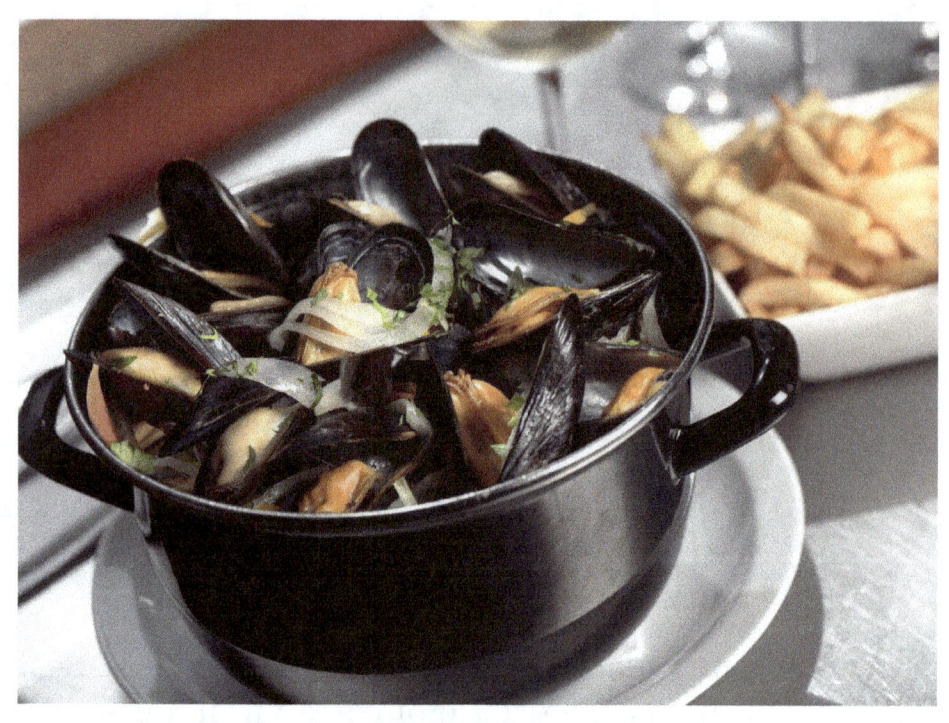

Mushroom Appetizer

Ingredients: 2 servings

- Fresh champignon mushrooms, 120 gr.
- Lemon, ½
- 2 anchovies in oil
- Capers, 1/2 tbsp
- Parsley, to taste
- Basil, 2 leaves
- Mustard, half a teaspoon
- Extra virgin olive oil, to taste
- Salt and pepper, to taste.

Directions:

1) Wash, drain and slice the mushrooms into thin slices. Arrange a chopped mixture with the cleaned anchovies, capers, basil and parsley. Add the mustard to the mixture and add some lemon juice to the mixture.

2) Season the sauce with extra virgin olive oil, salt and freshly ground pepper. Season the mushrooms with the sauce obtained. Stir and let it rest for 1 hour. Finally serve and enjoy your meal!

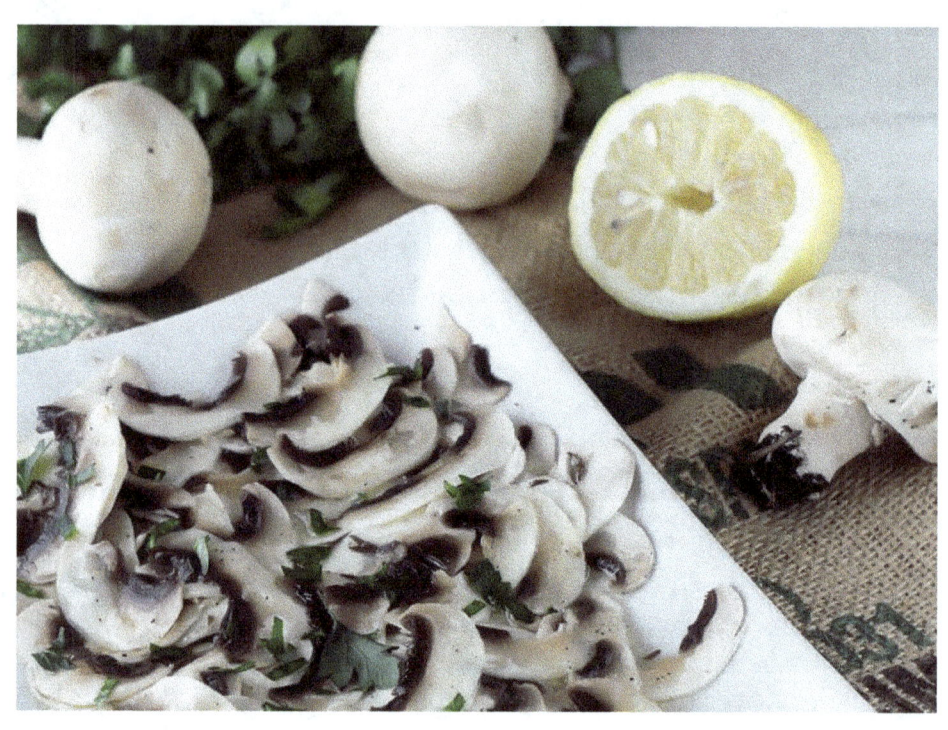

Anchovies with Lemon

Ingredients: 2 servings

- Clean anchovies, 180 gr.
- 3 untreated lemons
- Vinegar, to taste
- Oregano, to taste
- Extra virgin olive oil, to taste
- Salt, to taste

Directions:

1) Put the anchovies in a bowl. Put them under running water for half an hour until they lighten.

2) Take some vinegar and wash the anchovies. Put them in a glass dish. Sprinkle them with lemon juice and a pinch of salt. Leave them to rest in the refrigerator for four hours.

3) Remove them from the pan, clean the tail and season with extra virgin olive oil and oregano. Enjoy your meal!

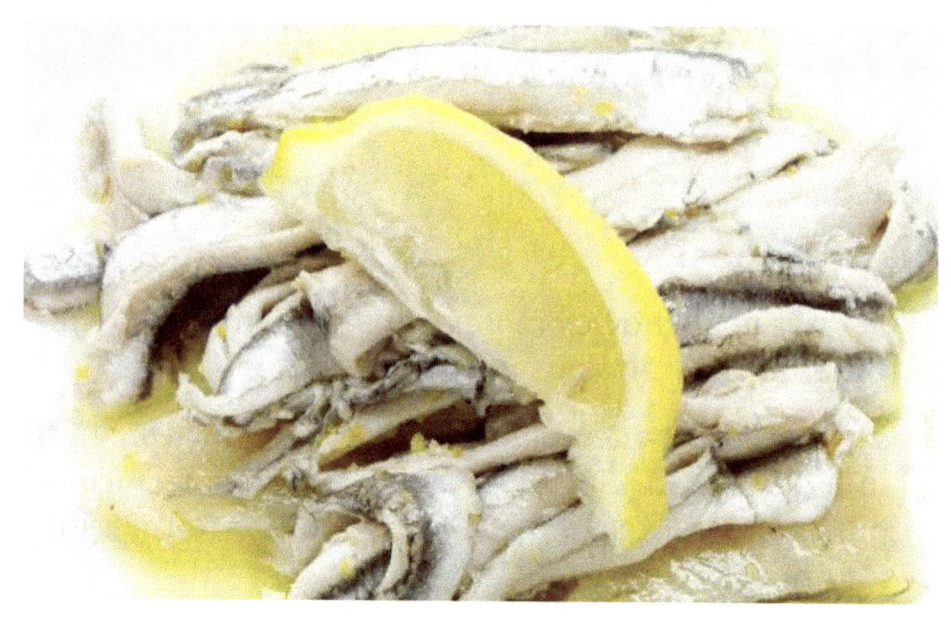

Sicilian Arancini

Ingredients: 2 servings

- rice, 100 gr.
- Peas, 100 gr.
- 2 eggs
- Butter, to taste
- Breadcrumbs, to taste
- Grated parmesan, to taste
- Onion, to taste
- Tomato paste, to taste
- Broth, to taste
- Seed oil, to taste
- Salt and pepper, to taste
- Chicken giblets, 50 gr.
- Ground veal, 30 gr.

Directions:

1) Cook a white risotto with butter. Add the grated Parmesan and 1 egg. Work the mixture.

2) Chop the meat and fry in a drizzle of oil. Combine the tomato paste. Extend with the hot broth. Season with salt. Add the peas and continue cooking.

3) Take the rice and make balls. Make a hole in the center where we will insert some sauce (ragù). Close the hole with rice. Beat the remaining egg and pass the rice balls over it. Put them in the breadcrumbs.

4) Fry in boiling oil, and drain them on kitchen paper to absorb excess oil. Serve hot. Enjoy your meal!

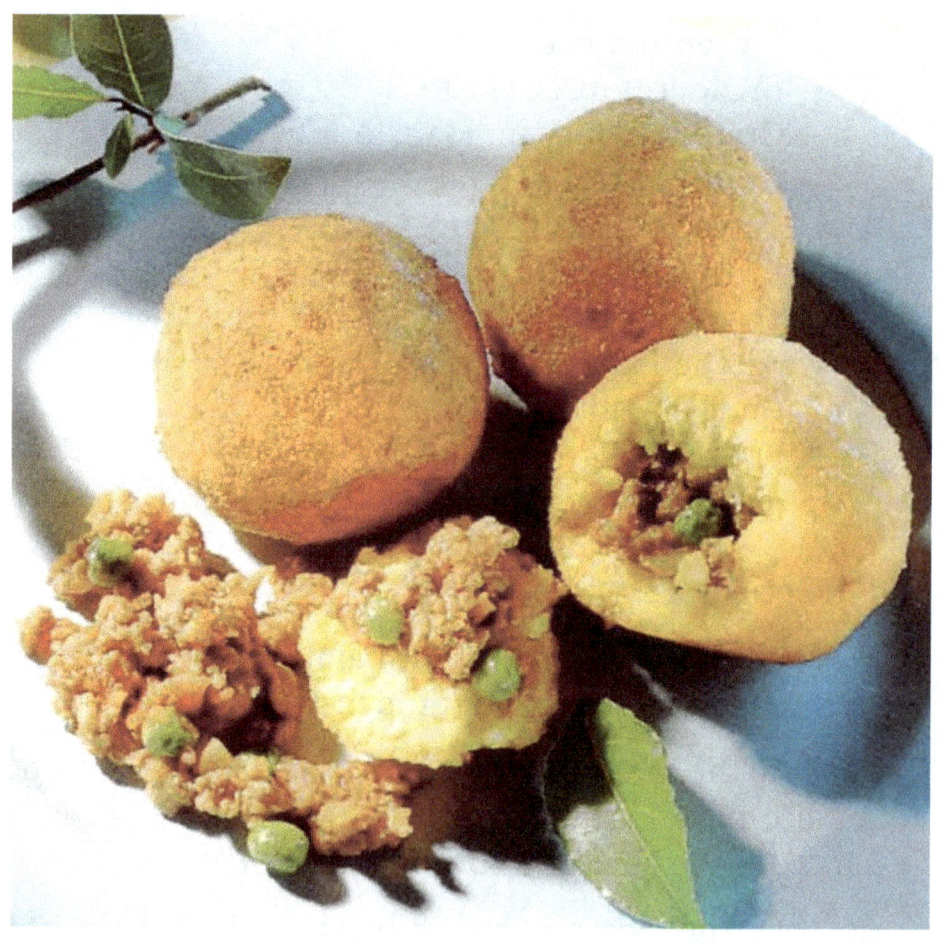

Cheese Puffs

Ingredients: 2 servings

- 6 small puffs
- Emmenthal, 20 gr.
- Sweet gorgonzola, 20 gr.
- Flour, 10 gr.
- Butter, 10 gr.
- Milk, 125 ml.
- 1 egg yolks
- Cream, 50 ml.
- Salt and pepper, to taste

Directions:

1) Heat the butter in a saucepan.

2) Incorporate the flour and mix in the roux. Extend with hot milk and cream. Stir until boiling. Season with salt and pepper.

3) Incorporate the diced sliced cheeses. Make it melt. Add the egg yolk. Work until you have a smooth and homogeneous mixture.

4) Fill a pastry bag with the appliance and stuff the cream puffs. Heat the oven to 180°C. and pass the puffs for five minutes. Serve hot and enjoy your meal!

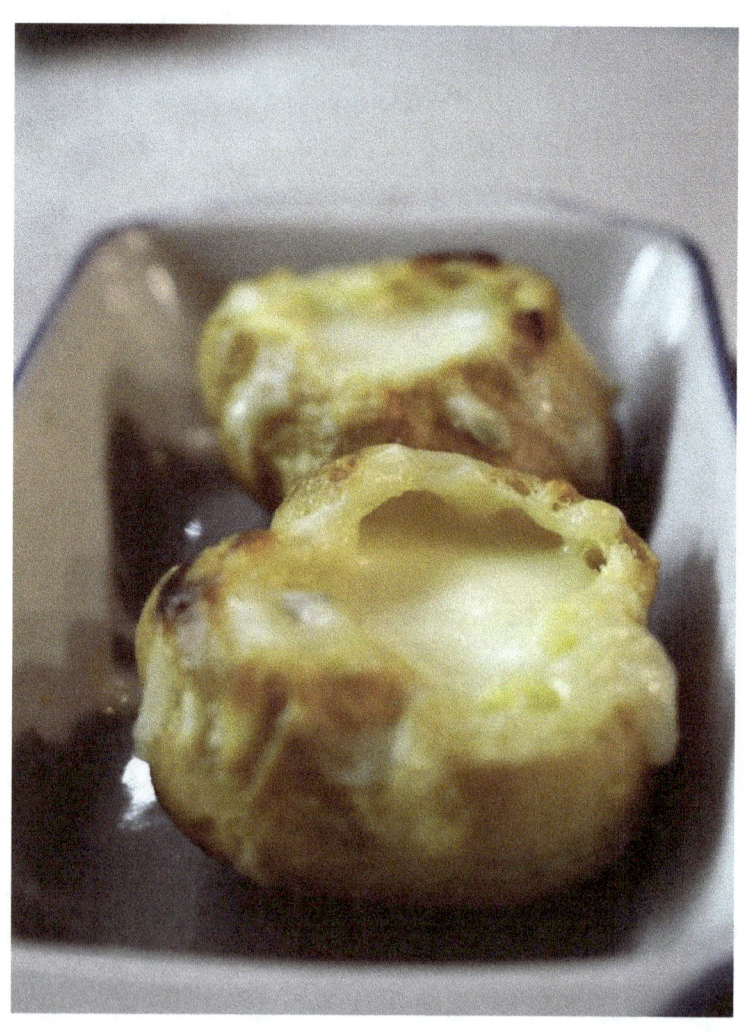

Ascolana Olives

Ingredients: 4 servings

- mixed ground (beef, pork, chicken), 250 gr.
- Lean raw ham, 50 gr.
- Mortadella, 3 slices
- Red onions, 1-2
- Medium carrots, 1-2
- Fresh parsley, 1 sprig
- Celery, 1 stalk
- Ground nutmeg, 1 pinch
- Breadcrumbs, 20 gr.
- 1 fresh lemon
- Extra virgin olive oil, 6 tbsp
- Soft wheat flour type 00, 20 gr.
- Salt and pepper, to taste
- Tomato paste, to taste
- Pitted green olives in brine, 300 gr.
- Olive oil for frying, to taste
- Grated parmesan, 3 tbsp

Directions:

1) Brown the coarsely chopped meats and vegetables in a pan with a little oil. Combine the concentrate diluted in a little warm water, add salt and pepper. The meat should not be fully cooked.

2) Then remove the vegetables and finely chop the mixture by adding ham and mortadella. Work the

mixture with the spices, a pinch of grated lemon zest, an egg, the chopped parsley, the wet and squeezed crumb, and the parmesan.

3) At this point, fill the olives with the mixture and give them a rounded shape. Then flour them, pass them in the beaten eggs and turn them in the breadcrumbs. Fry them in abundant boiling olive oil, remove excess oil by dripping them on absorbent paper, then serve them hot. Enjoy your meal!

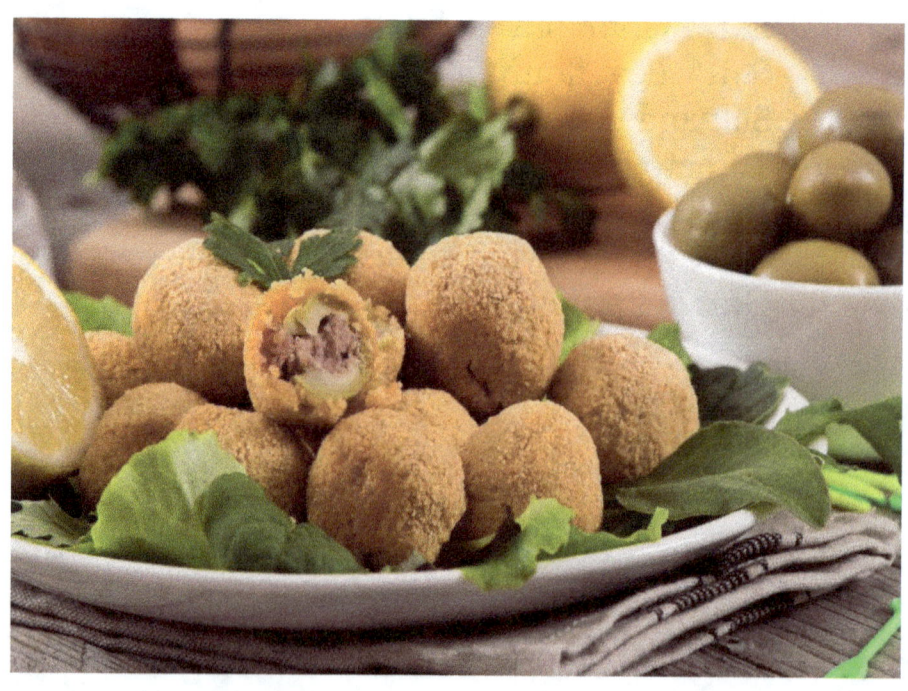

Broccoli Batter

Ingredients: 2 servings

- Broccoli, 500 gr.
- Re-milled flour type 0, 75 gr.
- Brewer's yeast, 5 gr.
- Butter, 10 gr.
- 1 egg
- Salt and pepper, to taste
- Vegetable oil for frying, to taste

Directions:

1) Cut the broccoli into small pieces. Boil them in salted water. In a bowl, work the flour with the yeast previously diluted with warm water. Combine the melted butter and salt. Incorporate the egg yolk while preserving the egg white. Let it rest for a few moments.

2) Resume and stir vigorously. Cover the bowl with a cloth. Allow about 60 min. Incorporate the whipped egg white.

3) Bring to temperature with oil in a frying pan. Dip the bits of broccoli into the batter. Dip them in boiling oil. Brown well. Drain them and spread them out on kitchen paper. Serve hot. Enjoy your meal!

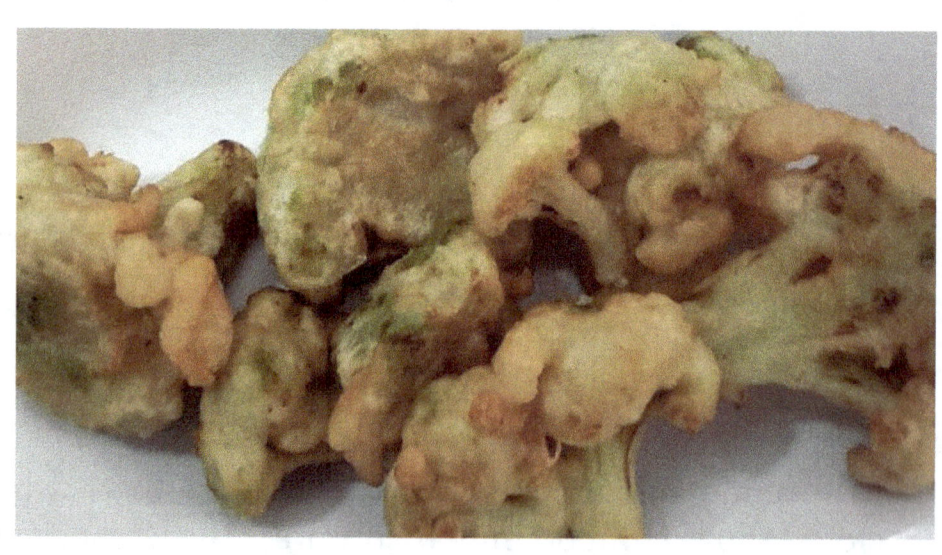

Baked Ham Croquettes

Ingredients: 2 servings

- Cooked ham, 4 slices
- Mashed potatoes, 200 gr.
- Mozzarella, 70 gr.
- Grated parmesan, 40 gr.
- Bechamel, to taste

Directions:

1) Season the mashed potatoes with the grated parmesan and the diced mozzarella.

2) Put a generous spoonful of the mixture on each slice of ham. Roll it up and close it with a toothpick.

3) Arrange the 4 croquettes in a lightly greased baking dish. Pour some bechamel over it. Put in the oven at 180°C for 20 minutes. Serve hot and enjoy your meal!

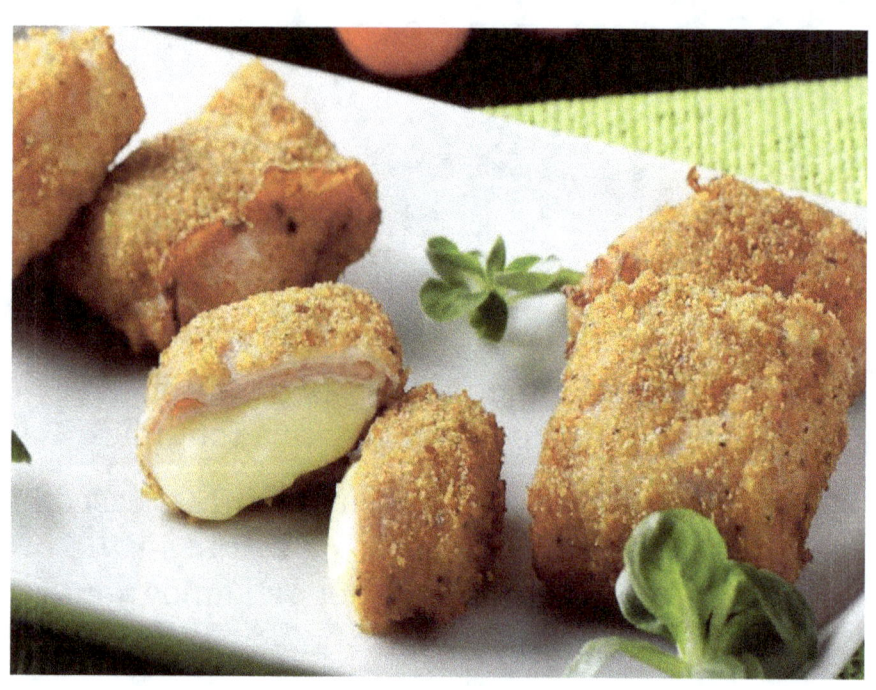

Cheese Patties

Ingredients: 2 servings

- Mascarpone cheese, 50 gr.
- Gorgonzola cheese, 50 gr.
- Stracchino cheese, 50 gr.
- 4 nuts
- Green peppercorns, ½ tbsp

Directions:

1) Mix the cheeses with the kernels of two walnuts. Work until you get a thick and homogeneous cream. Adjust with pepper.

2) Moisten two forms with water. Pour the mixture into the two forms. Level system and leave to rest for 3 hours in the refrigerator. Turn out the patties and garnish with the remaining kernels. Enjoy your meal!

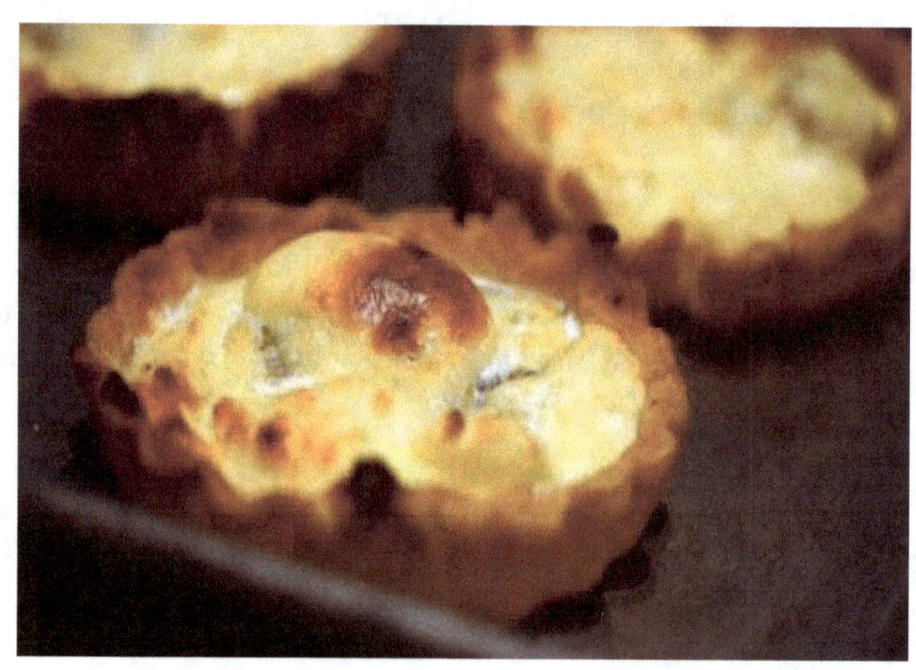

Main Courses

Cannelloni with Spinach

Ingredients: 2 servings

- Ready-made pasta, 220 gr.
- Spinach, 160 gr.
- 1 onion
- Garlic, 1/2 clove
- Green pepper, ½
- ground almonds, 60 gr.
- Thyme, 1 tsp
- Nutmeg, to taste
- 1 egg
- Extra virgin olive oil, to taste
- Grated Parmesan cheese, to taste
- Salt and pepper to taste

For the Tomato Sauce:

- Peeled tomatoes, 220 gr.
- Celery, 1 stalk
- 1 onion
- Garlic, 1 clove
- Chopped marjoram, to taste
- Tomato paste, ½ tbsp

Directions:

1) Prepare a sauté with chopped celery, onion, garlic. Pour in the peeled tomatoes and the tomato paste. Season with marjoram.

2) Close the pot and cook over low heat for about 20 min.. Stir every now and then in order to control the density of the sauce. Sear the spinach in boiling water for 2 min. Drain and squeeze them. Chop them up.

3) Brown a chopped onion and garlic with some oil. Add the spinach and cook. Clean the pepper by removing the seeds. Cut it into cubes. Add it to the spinach and cook for 5 min.

4) Bring the oven to 200°C. Mix the chopped almonds with the spinach. Lengthen with 150 ml. of water. Season with thyme and bring to a boil. Stir and season with a hint of nutmeg. Season with salt and pepper.

5) Roll out the dough and separate it into equal rectangles. Immerse them in boiling water for 2 min. in order to make the dough soft. Lever and dry. Fill with the spinach mixture. Brush the side with beaten egg yolk. Wrap and close well.

6) Butter a plate and prepare a tomato sauce base. Place the cannelloni and cover with the remaining sauce. Sprinkle with Parmesan.

7) Bake for 25 min. when the oven is already hot. Lever once au gratin and serve! Enjoy your meal!

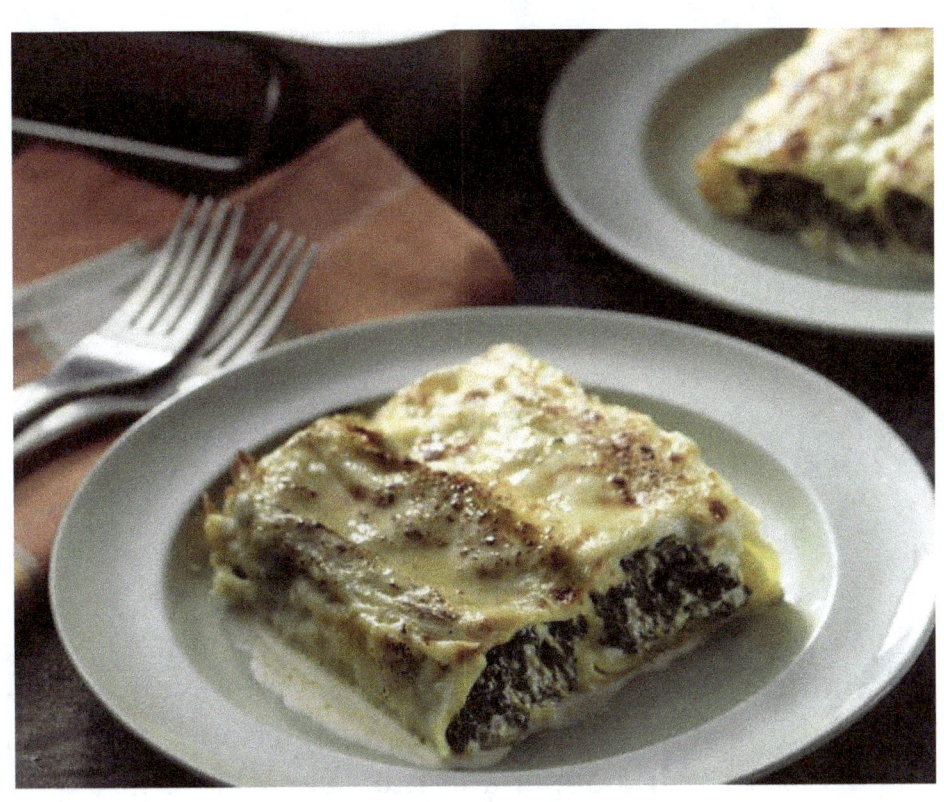

Pumpkin Tortelli

Ingredients: 2 servings

- Flour, 100 gr.
- 2 eggs

For the Stuffing:

- Pumpkin, 1700 gr.
- Amaretti, 30 gr.
- Parmesan cheese, 30 gr.
- Apple mustard, 30 gr.
- Nutmeg, salt, pepper to taste

Directions:

1) Prepare the pasta with the flour and eggs. Work it for a long time. Let it sit for 30 minutes.

2) Cook the pumpkin in a moderate oven for about 30 minutes. Let it cool down. Sieve it. Put it in a bowl. Combine the crumbled amaretti, chopped mustard, parmesan, salt, pepper and nutmeg. Mix well.

3) On a floured surface, roll the dough into a thin sheet with a rolling pin.

Cut it into small rectangles of about 8 x 4 cm. Put some filling. Close the bag rectangles by pressing firmly on the 3 sides with wet fingers. Boil the tortelli in abundant salted water for 5 minutes.

Season with melted butter and grated Parmesan cheese. Enjoy your meal!

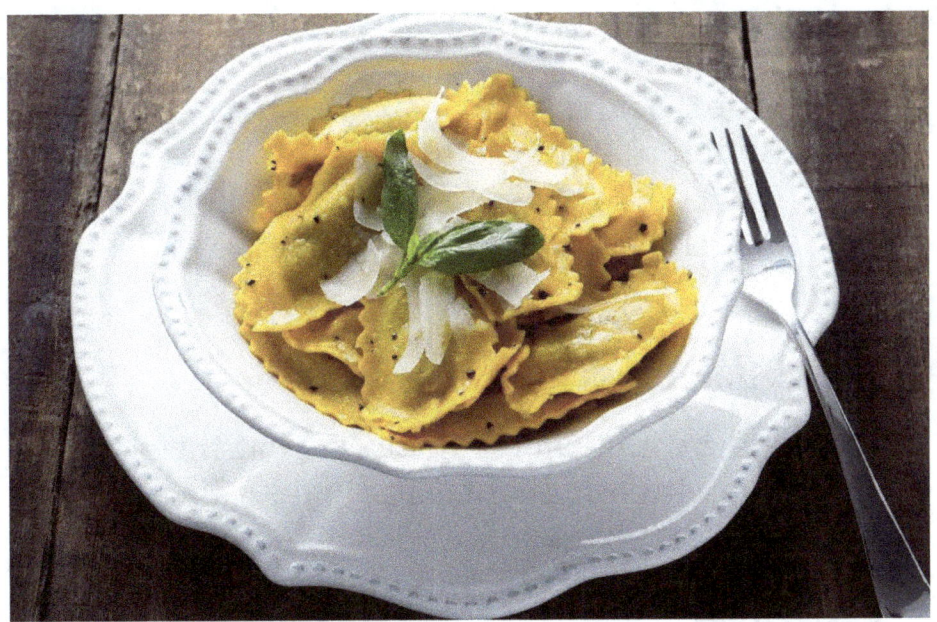

Timbale of Fusilli

Ingredients: 2 servings

- fusilli, 120 gr.
- 1 leek
- Dry white wine, 1 glass
- Milk, 1/4 of a glass
- Grated cheese, 40 gr.
- Egg, ½
- Sage, 2 leaves
- Butter, to taste
- Olive oil, to taste
- Salt and pepper to taste

Directions:

1) Slice the white part of the leeks. Put them in a small saucepan with a knob of butter and a finger of water. Over low heat, let them wilt slowly. Add the wine and let it evaporate. Pour in the milk and, always over moderate heat, let it be consumed. Adjust salt and pepper.

2) Boil the fusilli in abundant salted water and drain them. Butter a baking dish. Cover the bottom with a part of fusilli, arranging them so that they form a thick layer. Pour a little of the leek mixture on top. Sprinkle with grated cheese and flakes of butter. Make another layer of fusilli and another of seasoning, continuing this way until all the ingredients are used up.

3) Beat the eggs with a pinch of salt and a pinch of pepper, and pour them over the fusilli. Spread out a few more flakes of butter. Decorate with the sage leaves and bake in a preheated oven at 180°C for 40 minutes. Withdraw, let it rest for a while and serve! Enjoy your meal!

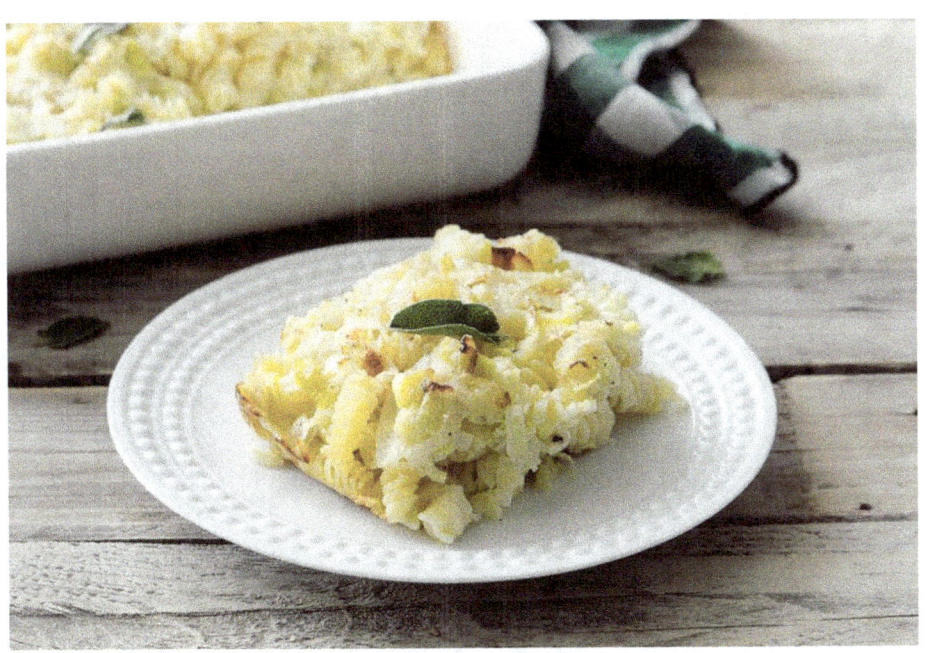

Orecchiette with Cauliflower

Ingredients: 4 servings

- Orecchiette, 400 gr.
- Green broccoli, 400 gr.
- Diced lard, 70 gr.
- Oil, 2 tbsp
- Grated pecorino cheese, 5 tbsp
- Salt, to taste

Directions:

1) Boil the broccoli. Drain and divide them into florets eliminating the hardest part.

2) Brown the lard with the oil and remove it from the cooking juices. Add the cauliflower and let it flavor. Cook the orecchiette, drain and toss in a pan with the cauliflower, add the lard and sprinkle with pecorino. Enjoy your meal!

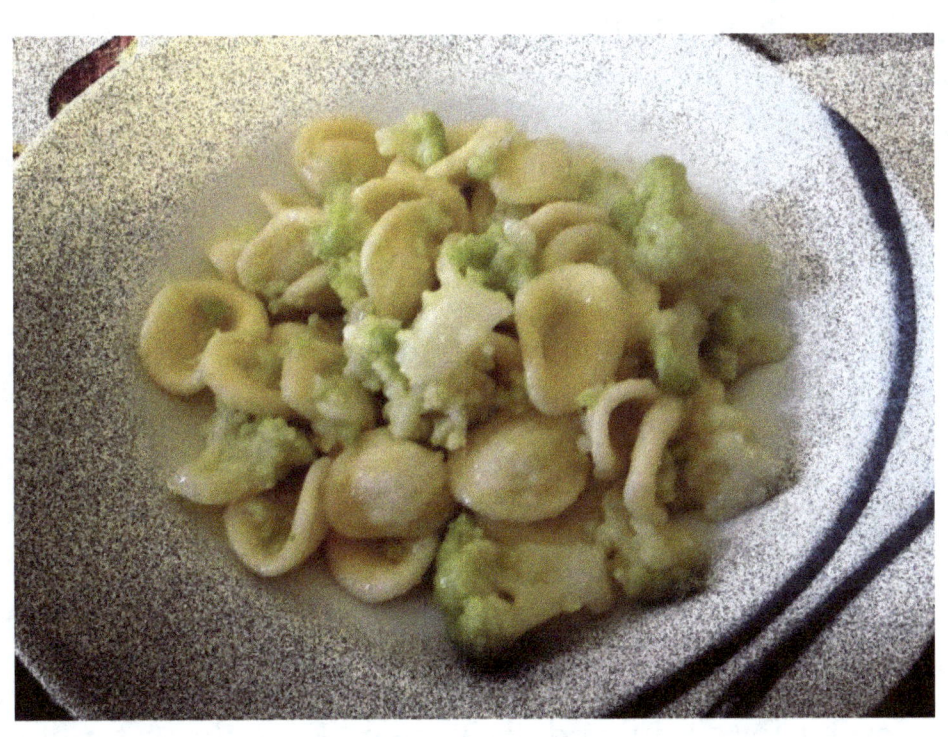

Macaroni with Artichokes

Ingredients: 2 servings

- macaroni, 160 gr.
- 3 Roman artichokes
- lemon, half
- Garlic, 1 clove
- Pitted olives, 60 gr.
- 1 hot pepper (of the red ones)
- 2 anchovies in oil
- Pickled capers, half a tablespoon
- Oregano, to taste
- Extra virgin olive oil, to taste
- Salt to taste

Directions:

1) Clean the artichokes. Eliminate hard leaves, internal hay, and tips. Chop them into wedges. Rub them with lemon so they don't blacken. Boil them in salted boiling water for 5 min. and drain them. Keep the water, it will be used to cook the pasta.

2) Fry the anchovies in a pan with some oil and garlic. Combine the olives without the pits. Add the julienned chili pepper. Combine the capers. Flavor with oregano. Let it flavor a few moments. Add the artichokes. Continue cooking for 10 min. on a low flame.

3) Cook the pasta. Drain it leaving it moist enough. Season it with the vegetables. Skip it for about 2 min. Season with pepper and serve. Enjoy your meal!

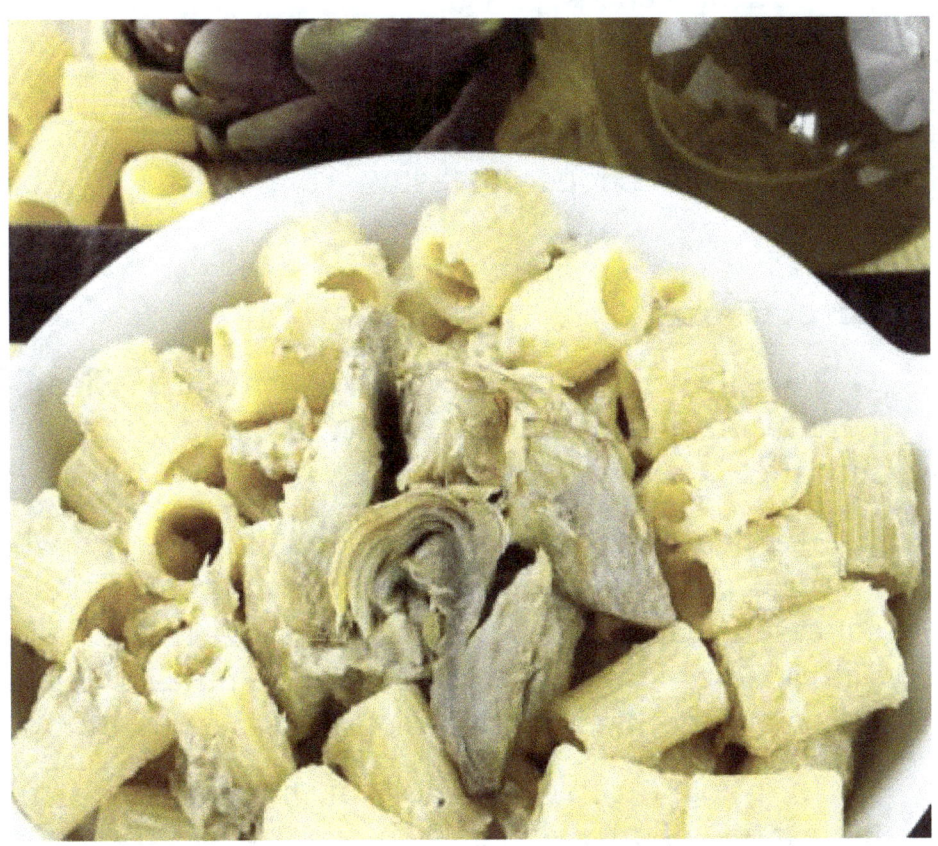

Farfalle with Mushroom Sauce

Ingredients: 2 servings

- Farfalle, 175 gr.
- Fresh porcini mushrooms, 100 gr.
- Dried mushrooms, 100 gr.
- Ricotta cheese, 25 gr.
- Tomato paste, to taste
- Garlic, to taste
- Olive oil, to taste
- Salt and pepper, to taste

Directions:

1) Soak the dried mushrooms in warm water. Clean the porcini mushrooms, chop half of them, cut the others into slices.

2) In a pan, heat three tablespoons of oil with a whole clove of garlic. Add the chopped mushrooms and the squeezed soaked ones. Let it dry, remove the garlic, wet with a ladle of water and cook for 20 minutes. Blend and mix the smoothie with the ricotta cheese.

3) In a pan, cook the porcini mushrooms with a tablespoon of oil, half a clove of garlic and a teaspoon of tomato paste, then mix. Add two tablespoons of water and cook for 15 minutes, salt and pepper. Boil the farfalle, season them with the ricotta smoothie and the sautéed mushrooms and serve. Enjoy your meal!

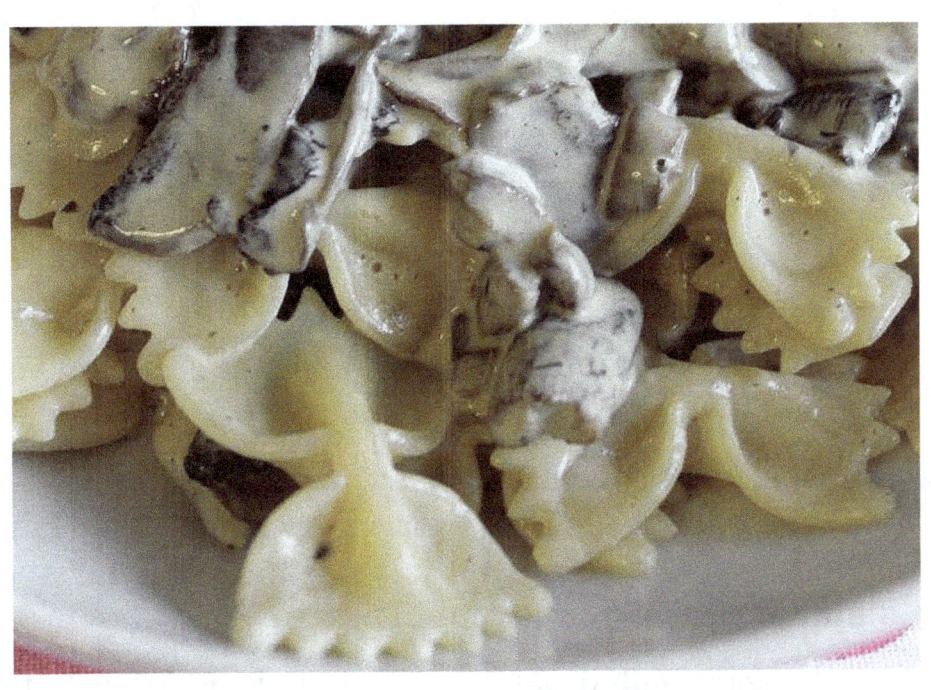

Fettuccine with Salmon

Ingredients: 2 servings

- Fresh fettuccine, 200 gr.
- Fresh salmon fillet, skinned and barbed, 100 gr.
- Yogurt, 1 tbsp
- Lemon juice, 1/2 tbsp
- Salmon roe, 1/2 tbsp
- Butter, 20 gr.
- Salt and pepper, to taste

Directions:

1) Chop the salmon fillet into small pieces and add salt. Season it with ground pepper.

2) Melt a piece of butter, not all of it, in a large pan which we will then use for the fettuccine. Combine the lemon juice. Add the pieces of salmon and cook for a few minutes. Turn around often.

3) Bring the salted water for the fettuccine to a boil, then throw the pasta. Combine the yogurt with the salmon. Make it warm up.

Mix the remaining butter and adjust the salt sauce. Drain the fettuccine and add them to the sauce. Blow them up for a few moments. Garnish with the salmon roe, and add the pepper. Place on the plate and serve! Enjoy your meal!

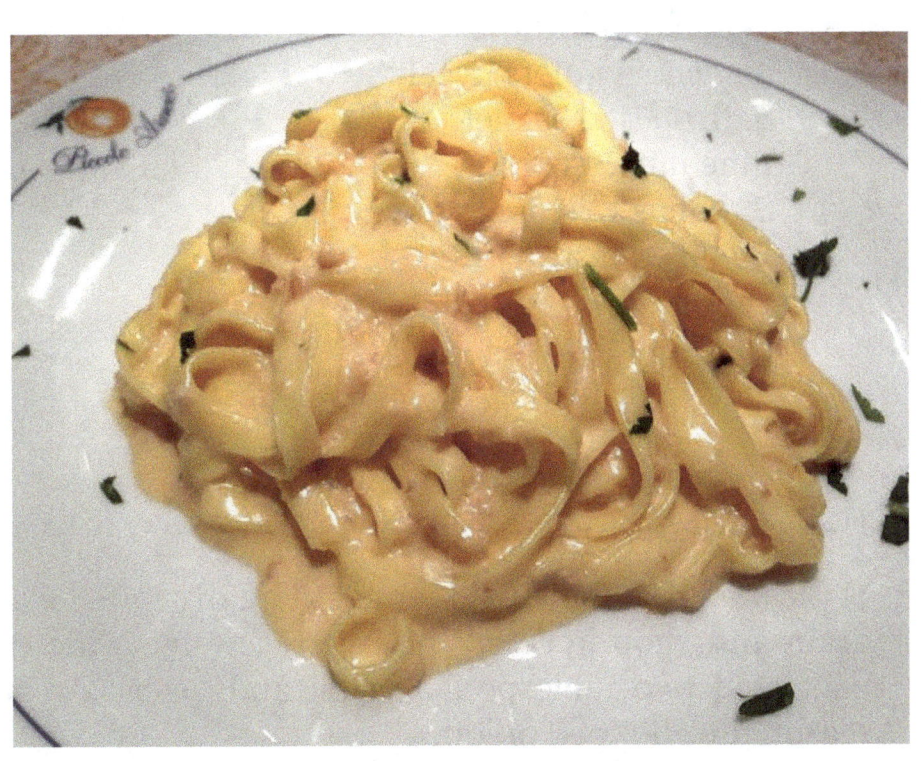

Pasta with Sardines

Ingredients: 2 servings

- Zite (pasta), 150 gr.
- Fresh sardines, 175 gr.
- Wild fennel, 100 gr.
- 2 anchovy fillets in salt
- Saffron, 1/2 sachet
- Pine nuts, 15 gr.
- Sultanas raisins, 15 gr.
- Flour, to taste
- Onion, ½
- Olive oil, to taste
- Salt, to taste

Directions:

1) Clean and boil the wild fennel in lightly salted water; drain and chop it. Keep the cooking water aside. In a pan, heat two tablespoons of oil and, over low heat, season the chopped onion.

2) Add the desalted and boned anchovy fillets and melt them. Then add the chopped fennel, the raisins softened in warm and squeezed water, and the pine nuts. Complete with the saffron, cover and cook over low heat for a quarter of an hour.

3) Open the sardines in half leaving them together along the back, clean them, wash them, dry them, flour them

and fry them in boiling oil. Drain them on absorbent paper and just salt them.

4) Boil the zite in plenty of water to which you added that of the fennel kept aside, drain and season with half of the sauce. Brush a pan with oil, arrange a layer of seasoned pasta and a layer of fried sardines on top. Sprinkle with a few tablespoons of the sauce and continue in layers finishing with the sauce. Place in a preheated oven at 200°C for 10 minutes and serve. Enjoy your meal!

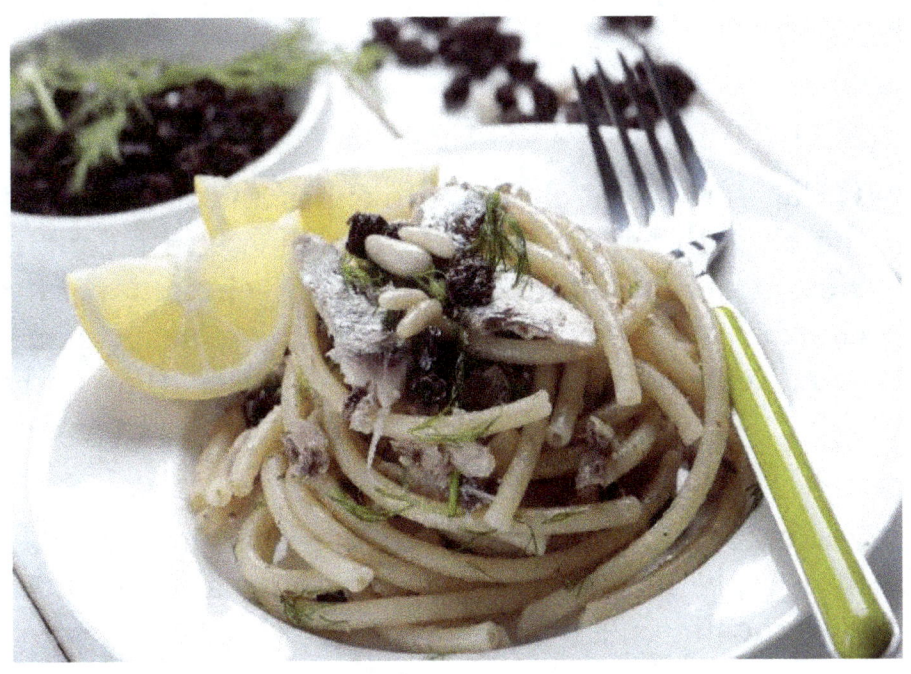

Rice with Peas and Cheese

Ingredients: 2 servings

- rice, 150 gr.
- Olive oil, 3 tablespoons
- Cinnamon, 1 stick
- Cardamom, 1 and ½
- Fresh chili, ½
- Cumin powder, 1 tsp
- Sugar, 1 tsp
- Peas, 150 gr.
- Low-fat cheese, 180 gr.
- Salt, to taste

Directions:

1) Cut the low-fat cheese into cubes and fry it in oil. Put the oil with which you fried the cheese in a container. Heat it and combine by mixing the cinnamon, cumin, chopped chili pepper; add the rice, peas, sugar then salt, cook, stirring constantly for 7/8 minutes, then add half a liter of water and boil. Cover and simmer for 20 minutes.

2) Remove the cover and add the fried low-fat cheese; mix gently, let it rest for a few minutes and serve. Enjoy your meal!

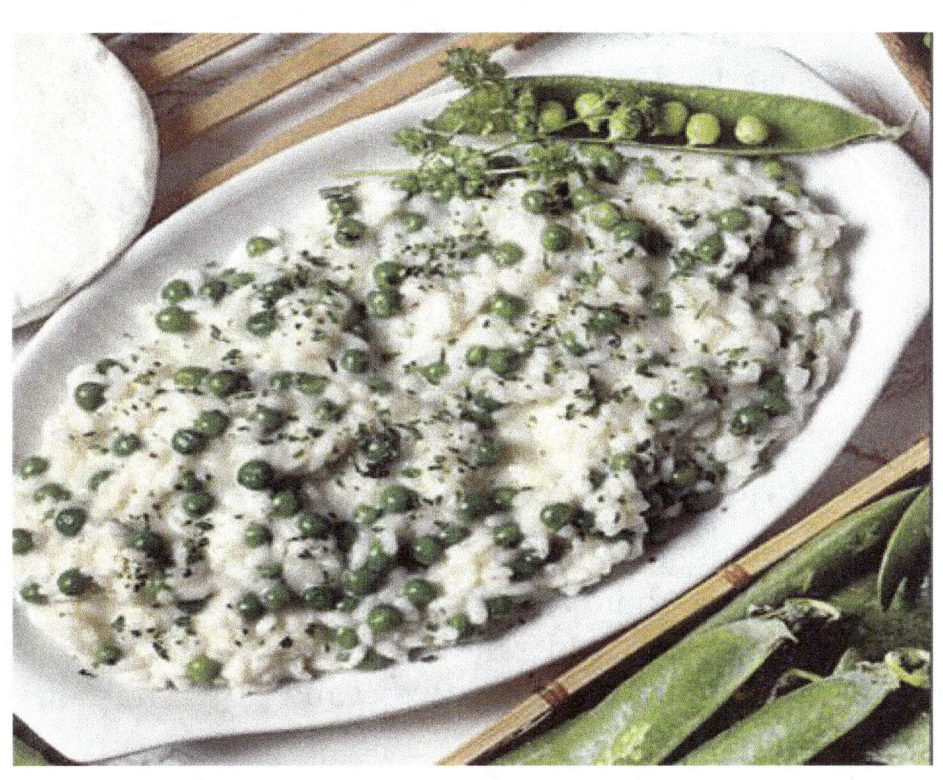

Mushroom Risotto

Ingredients: 2 servings

- 2 fresh porcini
- Rice, 160 gr.
- Chopped parsley, to taste
- Chopped onion, 2 tbsp
- Garlic, 1 clove
- Dry white wine, 1 glass
- Butter, 20 gr.
- Extra virgin olive oil, to taste
- Broth, 3.5 dl.
- Grated parmesan, to taste
- Salt and pepper, to taste

Directions:

1) Clean the mushrooms without rinsing them and chop them. Place them in a microwave-safe container with chopped onion. Add a drizzle of oil. Combine the garlic clove. Pour in the white wine and stir. Cook on full power for about 3 min.

2) Add the rice and pour in the boiling broth. Turn around and season with salt and pepper. Always cook at full power for about 15 min. Stir a couple of times during cooking. Finish and let it rest for 2 min. Stir in butter flakes. Sprinkle with chopped parsley. Season with grated Parmesan cheese. Enjoy your meal!

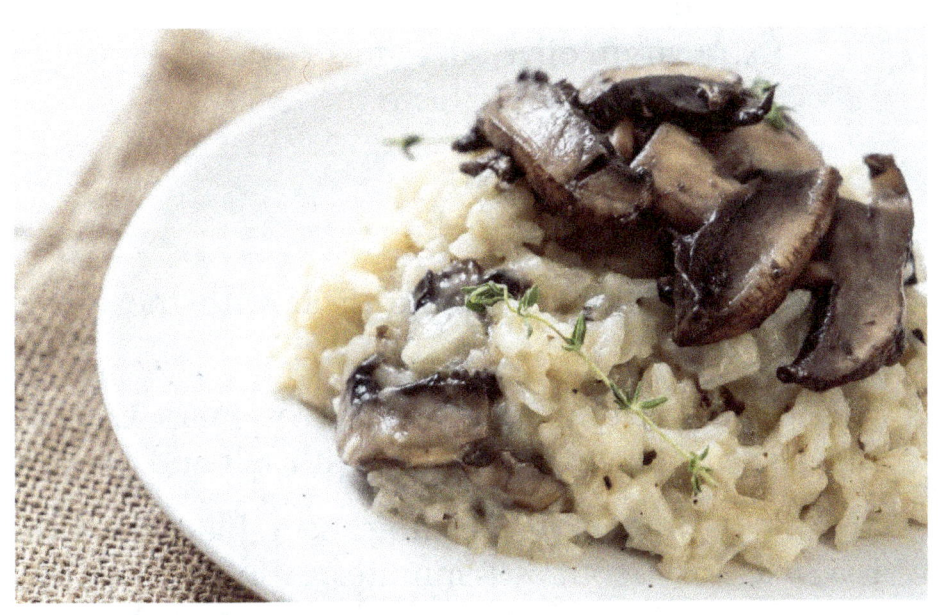

Baked Lamb

Ingredients: 2 servings

- Lamb, 450 gr.
- Bacon, 80 gr.
- Garlic, 2 small cloves
- Rosemary, 2 sprigs
- Extra virgin olive oil, to taste
- Salt and pepper, to taste

Directions:

1) Rinse the lamb. Stick the meat with the sprigs of rosemary.

2) Chop the garlic and add it to the rosemary. Cover with thin slices of bacon and season with salt and pepper.

3) Spread some oil on a baking sheet. Place the lamb in it. Bake for about 40 minutes, 180°C. Wet during cooking with the sauce you will get and serve. Enjoy your meal!

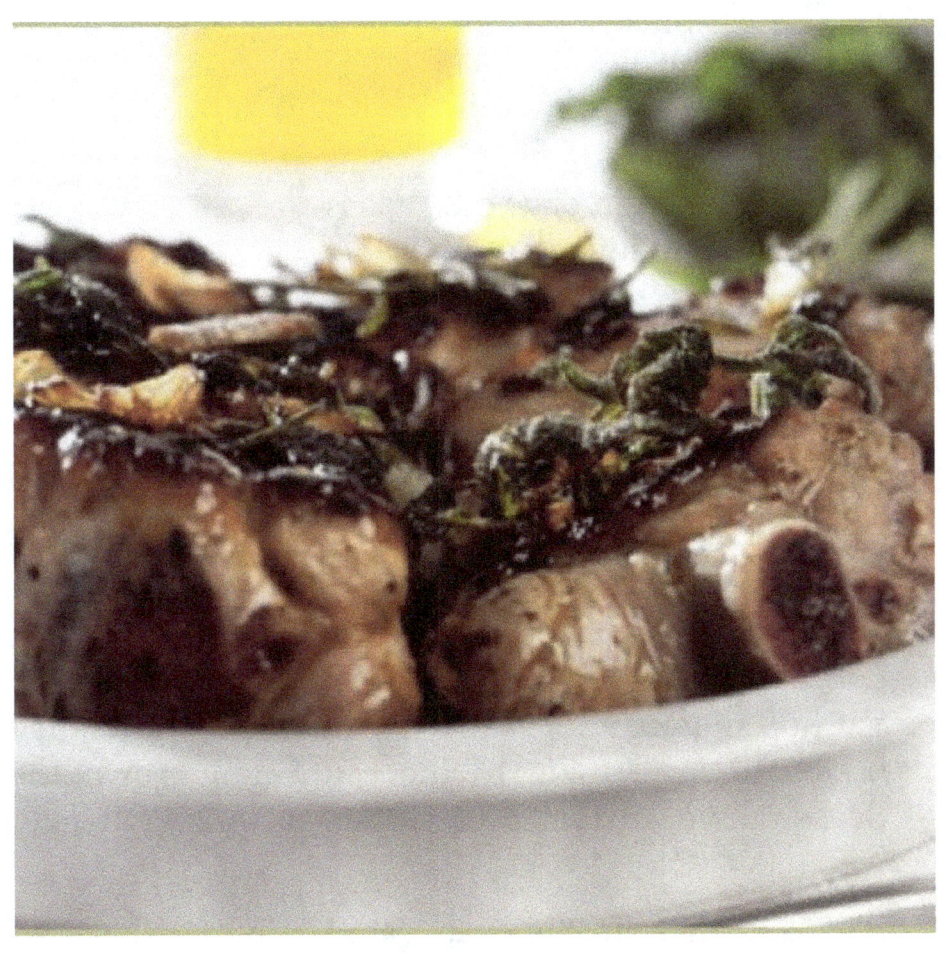

Ossibuchi with Mushrooms

Ingredients: 4 servings

- 4 ossibuchi
- 1 onion
- 1 carrot
- 1 celeriac
- Extra virgin olive oil, 1 glass
- Tomato pulp, 250 gr.
- Flour, 2 tbsp
- White wine, 1 glass
- Salt and pepper, to taste
- Garlic, to taste
- Rosemary, to taste
- Parsley, to taste

Directions:

1) Chop the vegetables and fry them with oil. Flour the ossibuchi. Add them to the sauté and brown them. Season them with salt and pepper, sprinkling them with wine.

2) When the wine is evaporated, pour in the tomato pulp. Cook for about two hours. Before removing them from the heat, add a mixture of garlic, rosemary and parsley. Serve them covered in a mushroom sauce. Enjoy your meal!

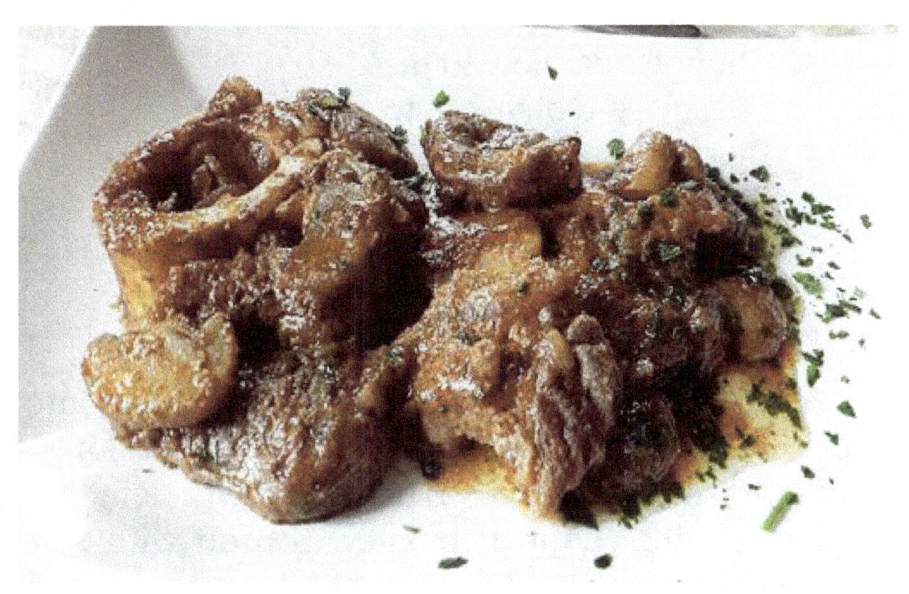

Turkey with Potatoes

Ingredients: 2 servings

- Turkey breast, 240 gr.
- 2 potatoes
- Lemon, ½
- Chopped parsley, to taste
- Extra virgin olive oil, to taste
- Broth, to taste
- Salt and pepper, to taste

Directions:

1) Peel the potatoes and rinse them; chop them into thin slices. Lay one layer on the bottom of a baking dish. Season with a drizzle of oil. Wet with lemon juice. Sprinkle with chopped parsley. Season with salt and pepper.

2) Arrange thin slices of turkey on top. Continue until you run out of ingredients. Sprinkle with broth. Close with transparent paper and prick it.

3) Cook for 14 min. approximately at maximum power. Let it rest for a few moments and serve. Enjoy your meal!

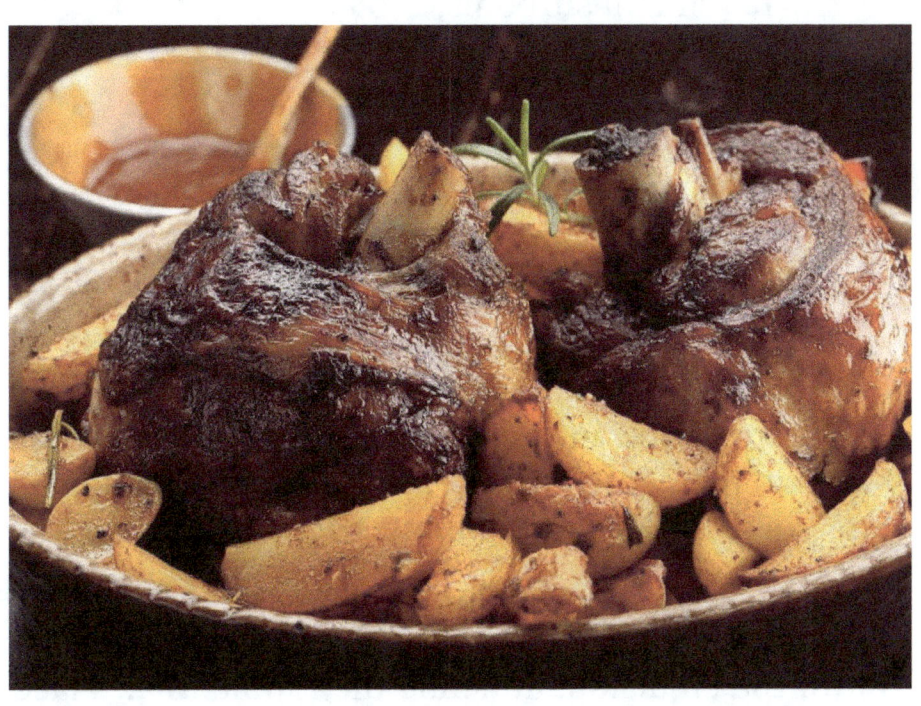

Beef with Mushrooms

Ingredients: 2 servings

- Fillet of beef, 220 gr.
- Porcini mushrooms, 130 gr.
- Emmenthal cheese, 30 gr.
- Extra virgin olive oil, to taste
- Parsley, to taste
- Lemon, ½
- Salt, to taste

Directions:

1) Chop the beef into small pieces. Clean the mushrooms and cut them into julienne strips. Place everything in the microwave. Cook for 2 minutes at a high temperature.

2) Emulsify some oil with lemon juice. Season with salt and parsley. Take the meat out of the oven and wet it with the emulsion. Julienne the Emmenthal. Place the cheese slices on top of the beef and serve! Enjoy your meal!

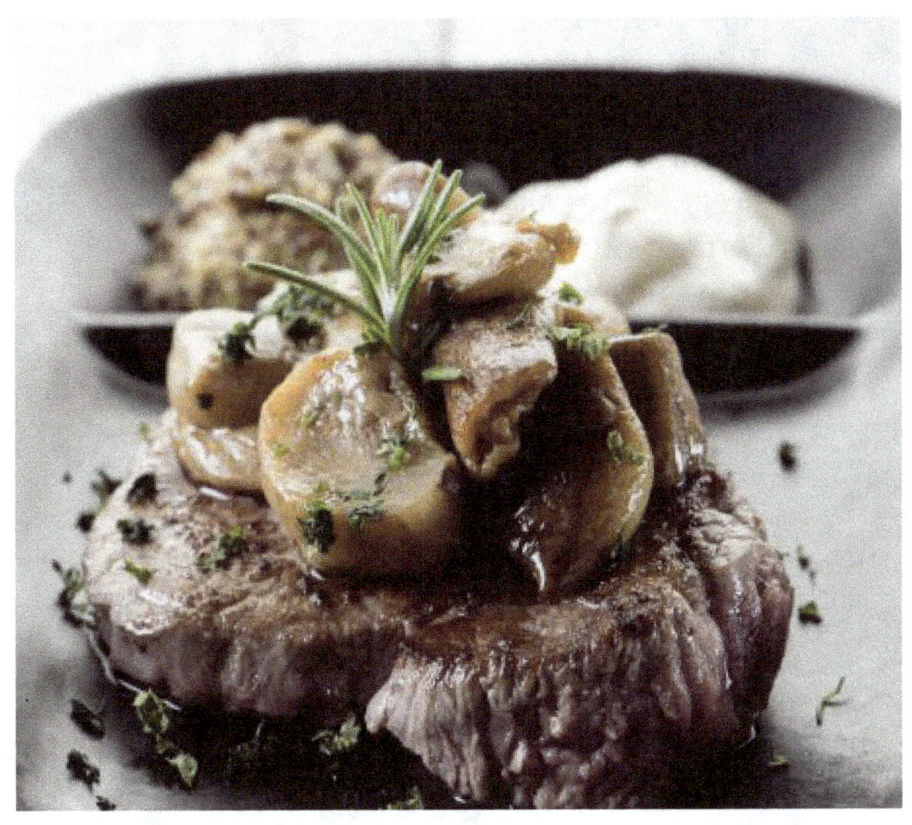

Pork with Corn

Ingredients: 2 servings

- Pork loin, 300 gr.
- Butter, 10 gr.
- Extra virgin olive oil, to taste
- 1 small onion
- Oregano, to taste
- Tomato puree, 200 gr.
- Canned corn, 125 gr.
- Hot chili, to taste
- Worcester sauce, to taste
- Salt, to taste

Directions:

1) Cut the pork into cubes.

2) Chop the onion and place it in a saucepan with the butter and a drizzle of oil. Combine the pieces of meat and brown everything.

3) Add the tomato puree and season with oregano; season with salt and pepper. Continue cooking for about half an hour.

4) Drain the corn and add it to the meat. Season with hot chili and 1 teaspoon of Worcester. Let it cook for a few more minutes and finally serve. Enjoy your meal!

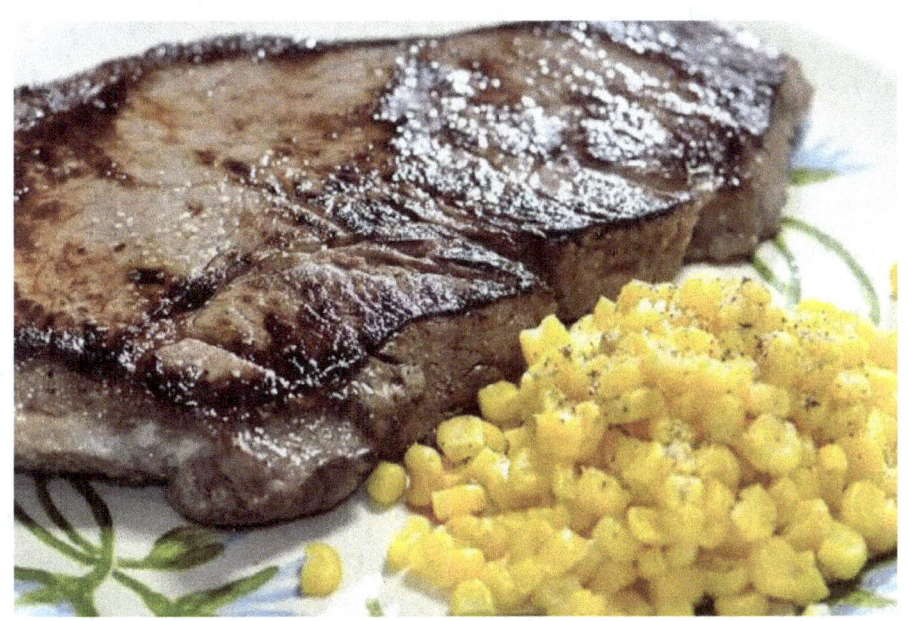

Cod with Lemon

Ingredients: 4 servings

- Desalted cod for at least two days, 500 gr.
- Extra virgin olive oil, to taste
- 1 lemon
- Parsley, to taste
- Garlic, to taste
- Black pepper, to taste

Directions:

1) Boil the cod for 10 minutes, then immerse it in cold water. Beat the oil with the lemon juice, the chopped parsley and the thinly sliced garlic.

2) Season the cod with the oil and lemon emulsion. Garnish with more parsley and black pepper. Serve warm or cold. Enjoy your meal!

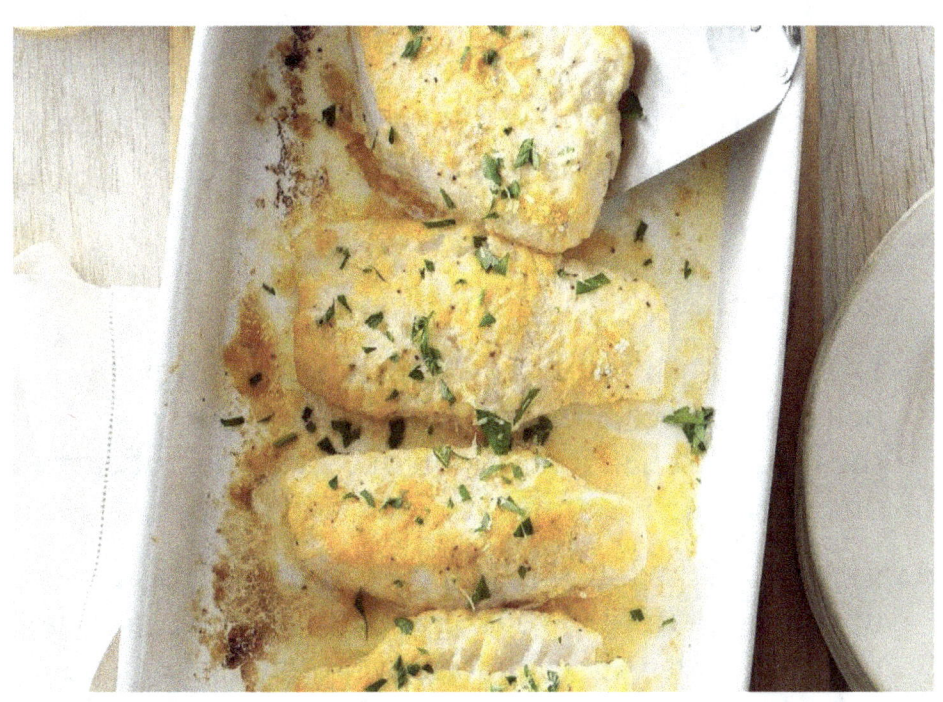

Lobster with Spices

Ingredients: 2 servings

- 2 frozen lobster tails
- Butter, 40 gr.
- Cilantro, 1 tsp
- Lemon, ½
- Ginger, to taste
- Curry, to taste
- Salt and pepper, to taste

Directions:

1) Thaw the lobster tails and cut the carapace on the belly. In a saucepan, just melt the butter, remove it from the heat, add half a teaspoon of ginger, half of curry and one of cilantro, lemon juice, salt and pepper.

2) Arrange the lobsters in a pan with the carapace facing up and cook in the oven for about 3 minutes, as much as possible under the grill. Remove, turn the tails, pour the spice butter into the central slot, place back in the oven for 3-4 minutes. Sprinkle with pepper and garnish with lemon slices. Enjoy your meal!

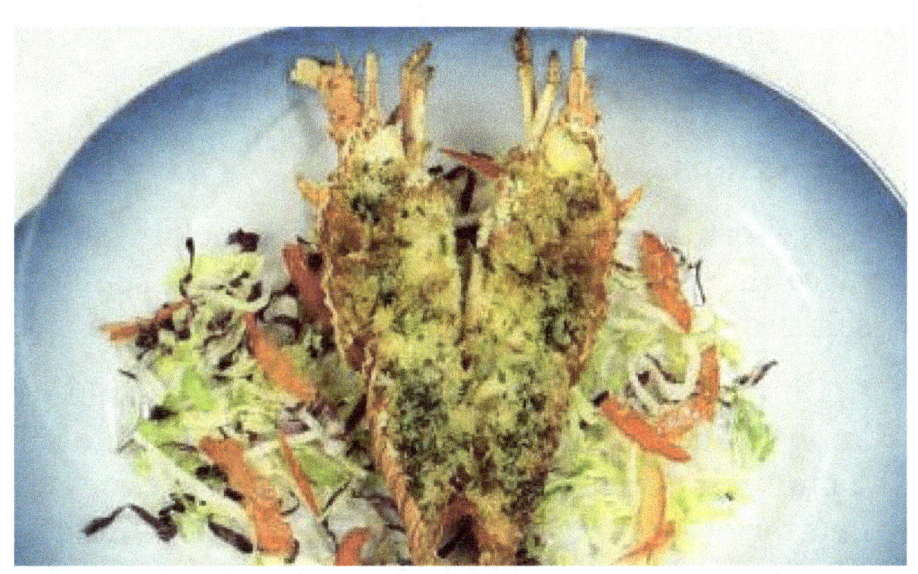

Trout and Nuts

Ingredients: 2 servings

- 2 trout already cleaned
- Walnut kernels, 100 gr.
- Butter, to taste
- White wine, 1 glass
- Sage, 4 leaves
- Cooking cream, 4 tbsp
- Salt and pepper, to taste

Directions:

1) Preheat the oven to 180°C. Grease a baking sheet and place the trout without overlapping them; season with salt and pepper. Sprinkle them with white wine.

2) Chop the walnut kernels. Sauté them in a pan with a knob of butter. Add the cream and let it bind for about 3 minutes. Spread it all over the trout. Bake for about a quarter of an hour. Sprinkle with a dash of milk while cooking and finally serve. Enjoy your meal!

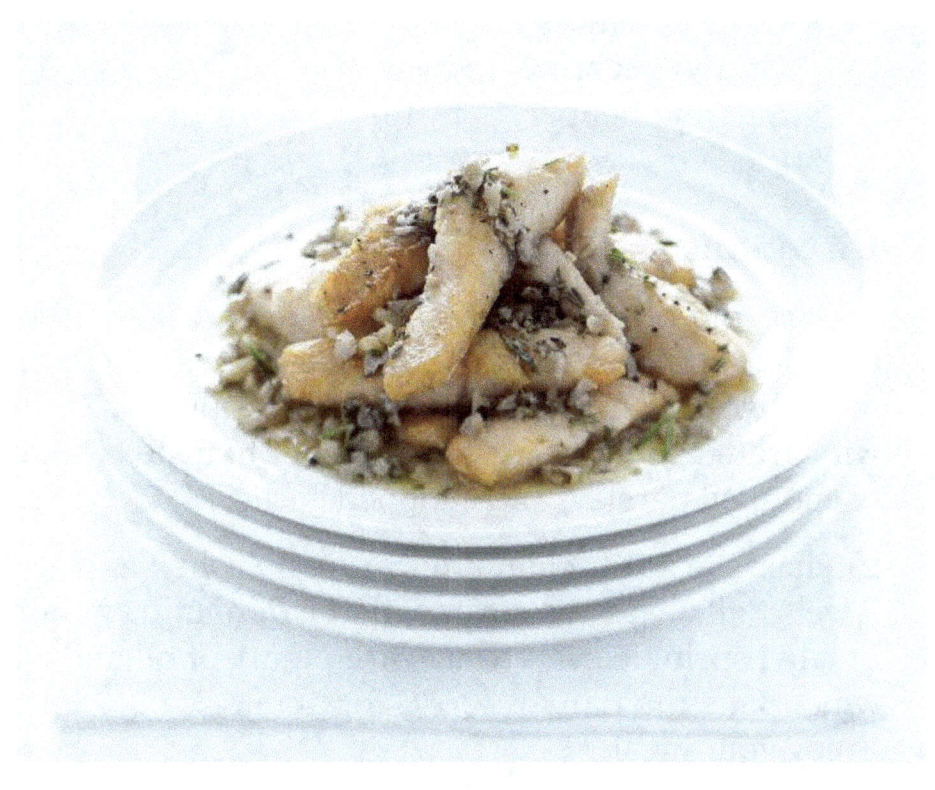

Sea Bream with Baked Potatoes

Ingredients: 2 servings

- 1 sea bream of 700-800 gr.
- 4 potatoes
- Chopped parsley, to taste
- Garlic, 2 cloves
- Grated pecorino, to taste
- Salt and pepper, to taste

Directions:

1) Slice the potatoes and soak them in cold water for about 20 minutes. In a baking dish, grease the bottom with olive oil, and cover with half the potatoes. Sprinkle with grated pecorino, salt and pepper to taste, a handful of chopped parsley, and chopped garlic.

2) Place the sea bream, after having washed and scaled it well. Salt again and cover with the remaining potatoes. Finally, sprinkle everything with plenty of oil and white wine. Bake the pan at 200°C for about 30-35 minutes. Enjoy your meal!

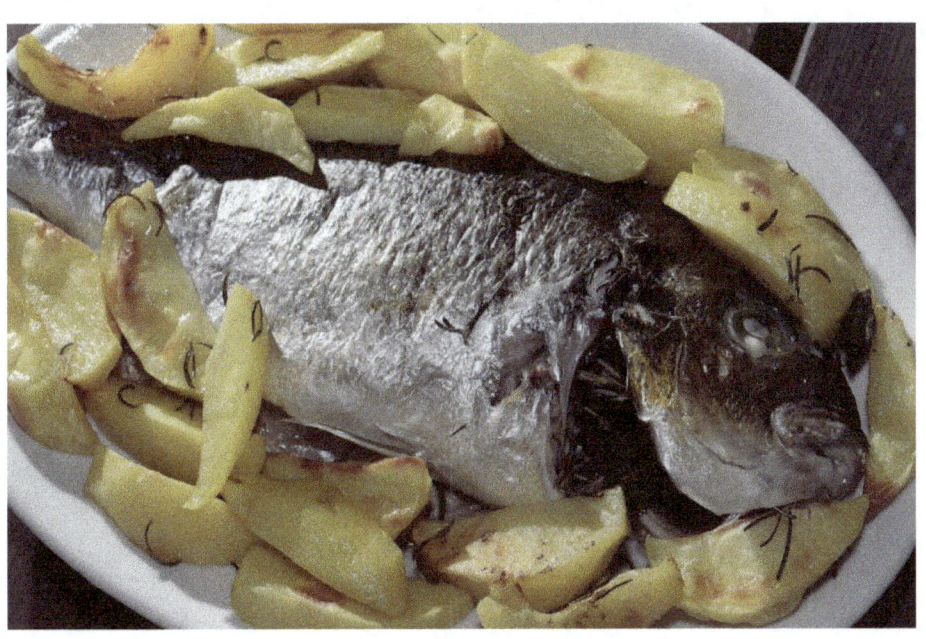

Perch with Cherry Tomatoes and Basil

Ingredients: 2 servings

- Perch fillets, 300 gr.
- Tomatoes, 2 medium-sized
- Extra virgin olive oil, to taste
- White wine, 1 glass
- Chopped basil, to taste

Directions:

1) Cut the tomatoes into small cubes. Heat a little oil in a saucepan.

2) Add the cleaned perch fillets. Brown them on both sides and add the tomatoes. Wet with white wine; season with salt and pepper. Season with plenty of chopped basil. Cook and serve. Enjoy your meal!

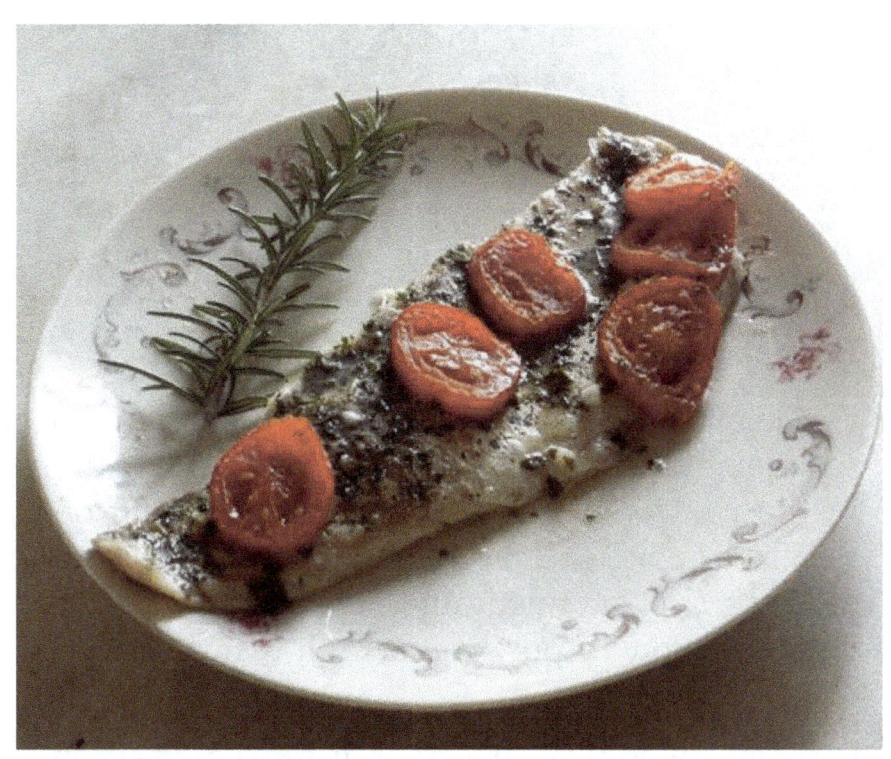

Side Dishes

Parmigiana Asparagus

Ingredients: 2 servings

- Asparagus tips, 300 gr.
- Raw ham, 2 slices
- Grated parmesan cheese, 40 gr.
- Cream, 2 tbsp
- Salt and pepper, to taste

Directions:

1) Clean the asparagus so they are ready to cook. Arrange them in a radial pattern on a plate with the tips in the center. Wet them with 1 tablespoon of water. Cover the plate with cling paper. Cook them for 6 min. approximately at maximum power. Turn the asparagus halfway through cooking and let it rest for a moment.

2) Move the asparagus to a Pyrex container lined up next to each other. Season with salt and pepper. Place the slices of raw ham on top. Season with grated Parmesan cheese and spread some cream. Cook uncovered for about 1 min. Serve hot and au gratin. Enjoy your meal!

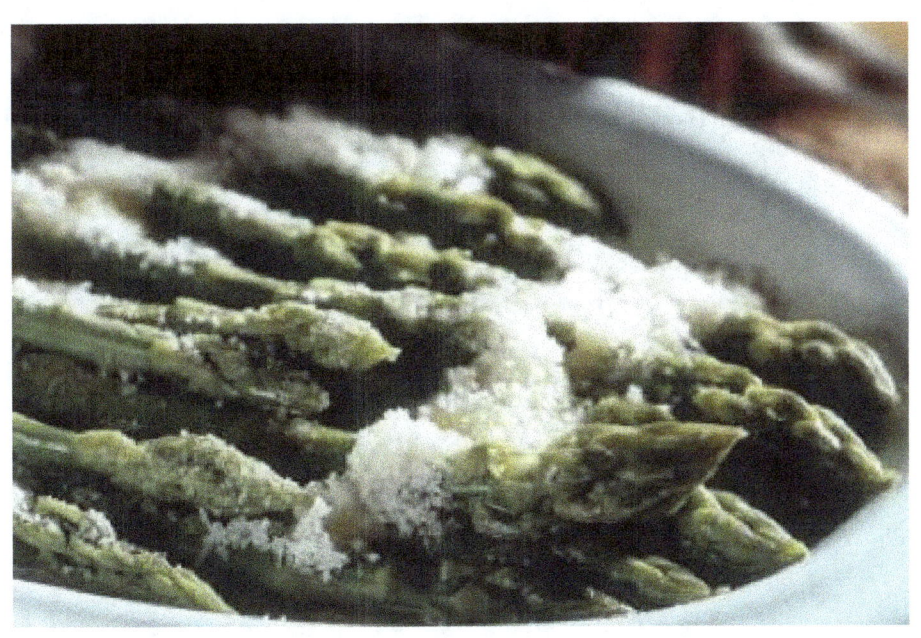

Piemontese Polenta

Ingredients: 2 servings

- Corn flour, 250 gr.
- White flour, 50 gr.
- Fontina cheese from Valle d'Aosta, 150 gr.
- Grated Parmesan cheese, 100 gr.
- Butter, 50 gr.
- Vegetable broth, 1/2 l.
- Partially skimmed milk, 1 glass
- Liquid cream, 200 ml.
- 1 white onion
- 1 medium leek
- Celery, 1 stalk
- Fresh garlic, 2 cloves
- Sage, to taste
- Fresh rosemary, 1 sprig
- Fresh basil, to taste
- Bay leaf, 1 leaf
- Extra virgin olive oil, 3 tbsp
- Salt and pepper, to taste

Directions:

1) Put the broth and milk in a saucepan and bring them to a boil. Mix the two types of flour together. Scrape the celery stalk, peel the onion and garlic and clean the leek; then chop everything together, pour it into a bowl and mix the oil.

2) Put the mince to brown in a pan over medium heat and, when everything is well wilted, remove it from the heat. As soon as the broth and milk have reached a boil, pour in the mixed flours and cook for about half an hour. Stir constantly with a wooden spoon, so that no lumps form.

3) At the end of cooking, mix the sautéed, diced fontina cheese, butter, cream, salt and pepper with the polenta and remove from heat. Clean and wash the sage, rosemary, basil and bay leaf and chop them together. Combine them with the polenta together with the Parmesan cheese, whisk and serve hot. Enjoy your meal!

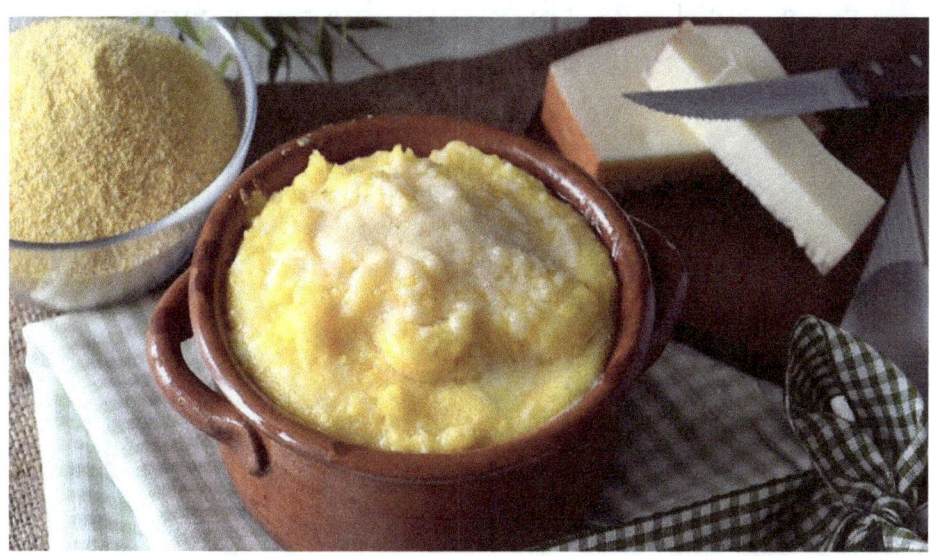

Carrot Puree

Ingredients: 2 servings

- Clean carrots, 160 gr.
- Sugar, 1 tsp
- Butter, 20 gr.
- Liquid cream, 2 tbsp
- Salt, to taste

Directions:

1) Chop the carrots. Cook them in water with salt, sugar and half butter. Remove them once cooked. Drain them, pass them to the mixer, and place in a pan.

2) Add the remaining butter and season with salt. Stir over a low flame. Thicken the heated cream a little at a time. Work and remove once you have a smooth and fluffy mixture. Serve. Enjoy your meal!

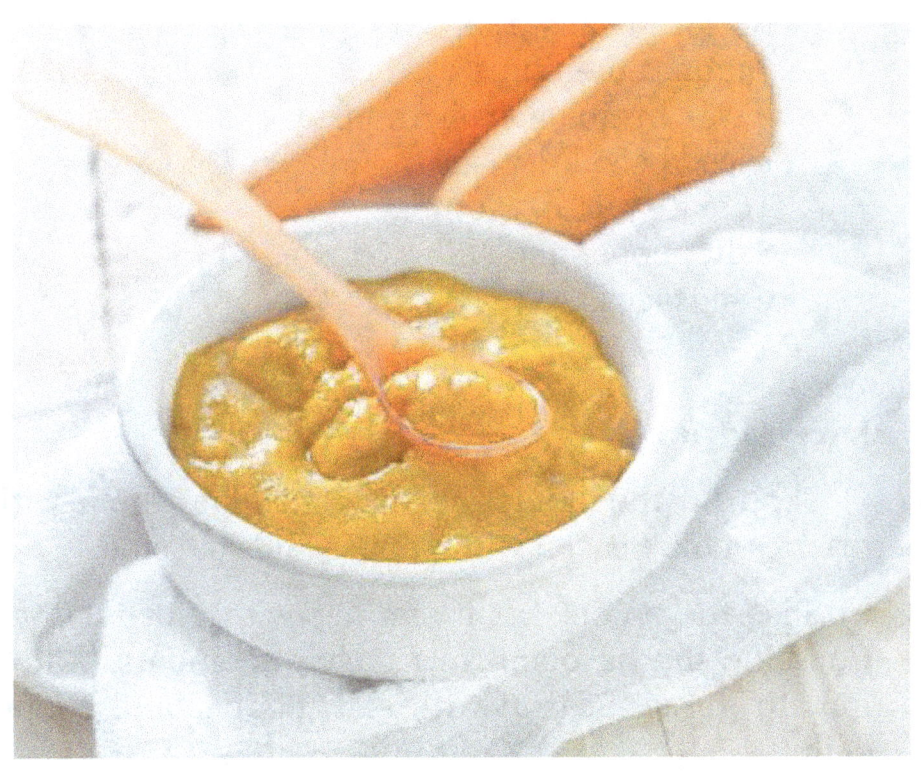

Mexican Beans

Ingredients: 2 servings

- Borlotti beans, 1 box
- Onion, 1 medium
- Extra virgin olive oil, to taste
- Diced bacon, 100 gr.
- Tomato puree, 150 ml.
- Salt, pepper and chili, to taste
- 2 sausages

Directions:

1) Chop up the skinless sausages. Sauté them with a drizzle of oil. Season with pepper and set aside.

2) Slice the onion. Let it simmer with a drizzle of oil. Combine the bacon. Brown a few moments. Add the tomato puree. Season with salt, pepper and chopped chili.

3) Now mix the beans. Dilute the beans with a drop of cooking water. Cook on a gentle flame. Add the sausages and finish cooking. Serve. Enjoy your meal!

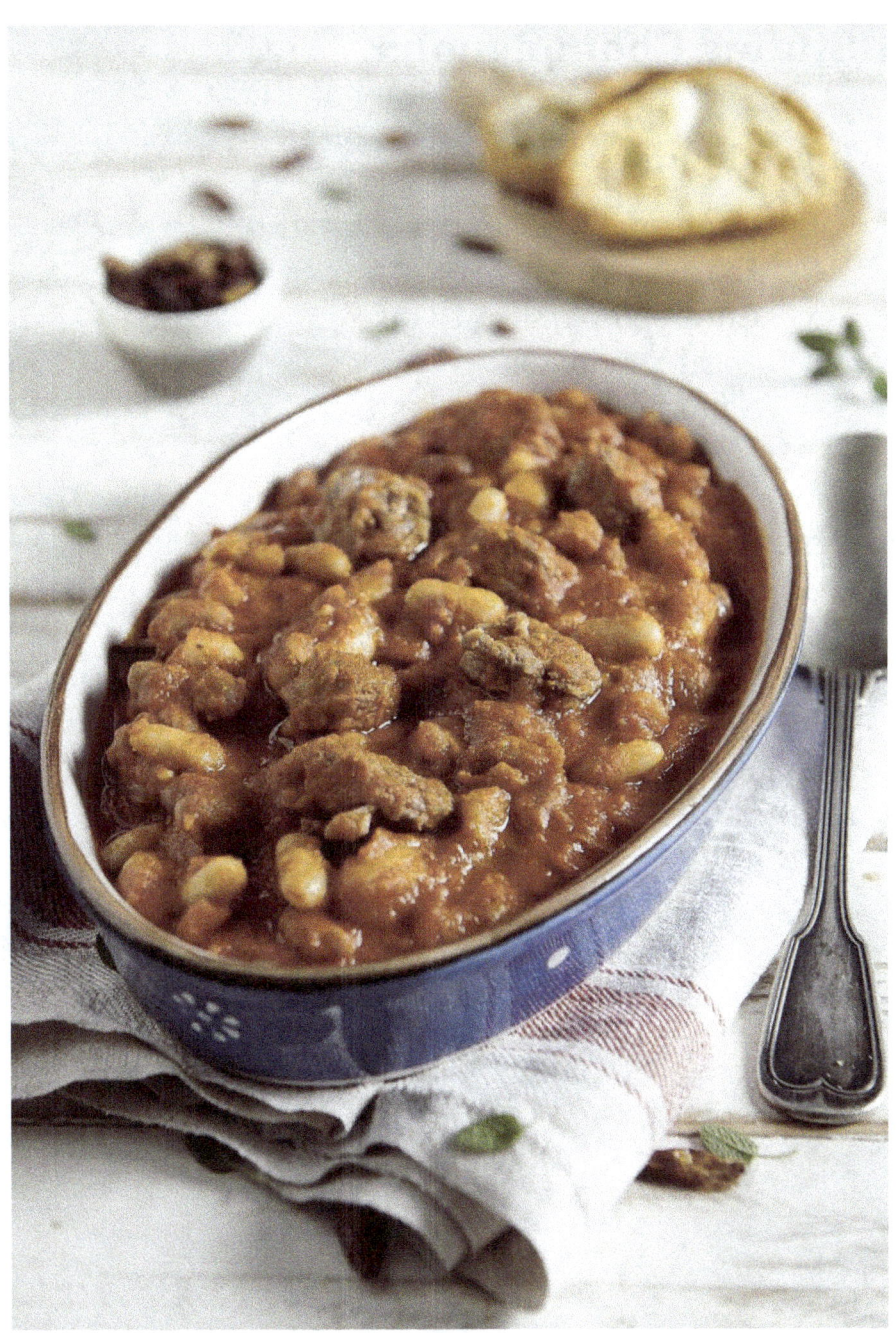

Stuffed Champignons

Ingredients: 2 servings

- Champignons chapels, 125 gr.
- Extra virgin olive oil, 15 gr.
- Chopped parsley, to taste
- Garlic, 1 clove
- Salt and pepper, to taste

Directions:

1) Clean the caps of the mushrooms.

2) Put them in the microwave for 2 minutes on a serving dish, covered with the oil, the chopped parsley and the garlic. Uncover them, salt them lightly and let them rest for 1 minute before serving. Enjoy your meal!

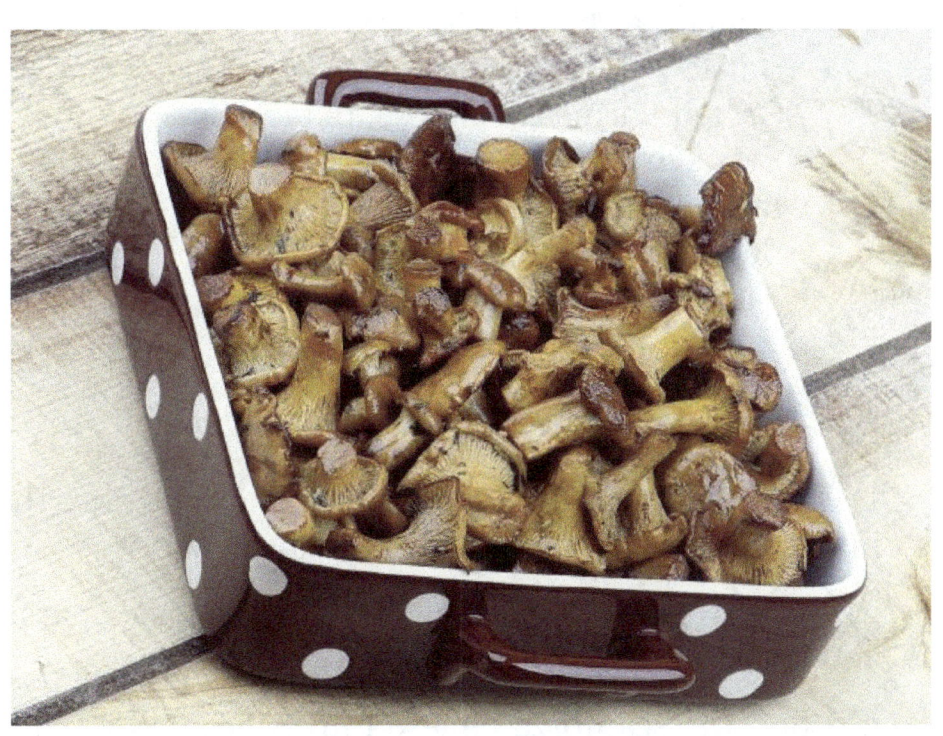

Baked Zucchini

Ingredients: 2 servings

- Zucchini, 280 gr.
- Diced tomato pulp, 120 gr.
- Scamorza cheese, 160 gr.
- Garlic
- Grated Parmesan cheese, to taste
- Extra virgin olive oil, to taste
- Butter, 30 gr.
- Basil and parsley, to taste
- Salt and pepper, to taste

Directions:

1) Clean the zucchini. Remove both ends and slice them into long slices. Blanch in boiling salted water.

2) Clean the parsley. Prepare chopped basil, parsley, and garlic.

3) Chop the scamorza cheese into cubes. Oil a plaque. Make a layer of zucchini. Sprinkle with chopped herbs. Season with salt and pepper.

4) Place a few tablespoons of tomato cubes. Sprinkle with grated Parmesan cheese. Put some cubes of smoked cheese. Sprinkle a little oil. Continue these operations until the ingredients are finished. Finally, deposit the knobs of butter. Bake for 20 min. at 180°C. Serve. Enjoy your meal!

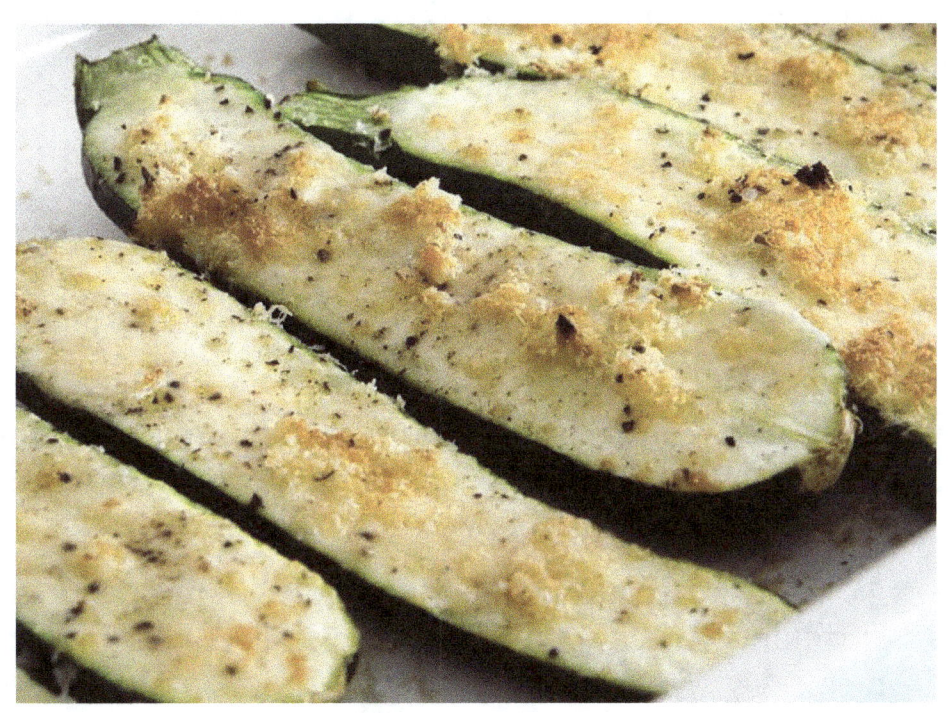

Sautéed Mushrooms

Ingredients: 2 servings

- Porcini mushrooms, 360 gr.
- Extra virgin olive oil, to taste
- Garlic, 1 clove
- Chopped parsley, to taste
- Salt and pepper, to taste
- White wine, to taste

Directions:

1) Clean the mushrooms and cut them into julienne strips.

2) Fry the garlic. Add the mushrooms and let them flavor. Wet with a drop of wine and let it evaporate. Season with salt and pepper.

3) Cook on a moderate flame for 30 min. Stir and sprinkle with chopped parsley and serve. Enjoy your meal!

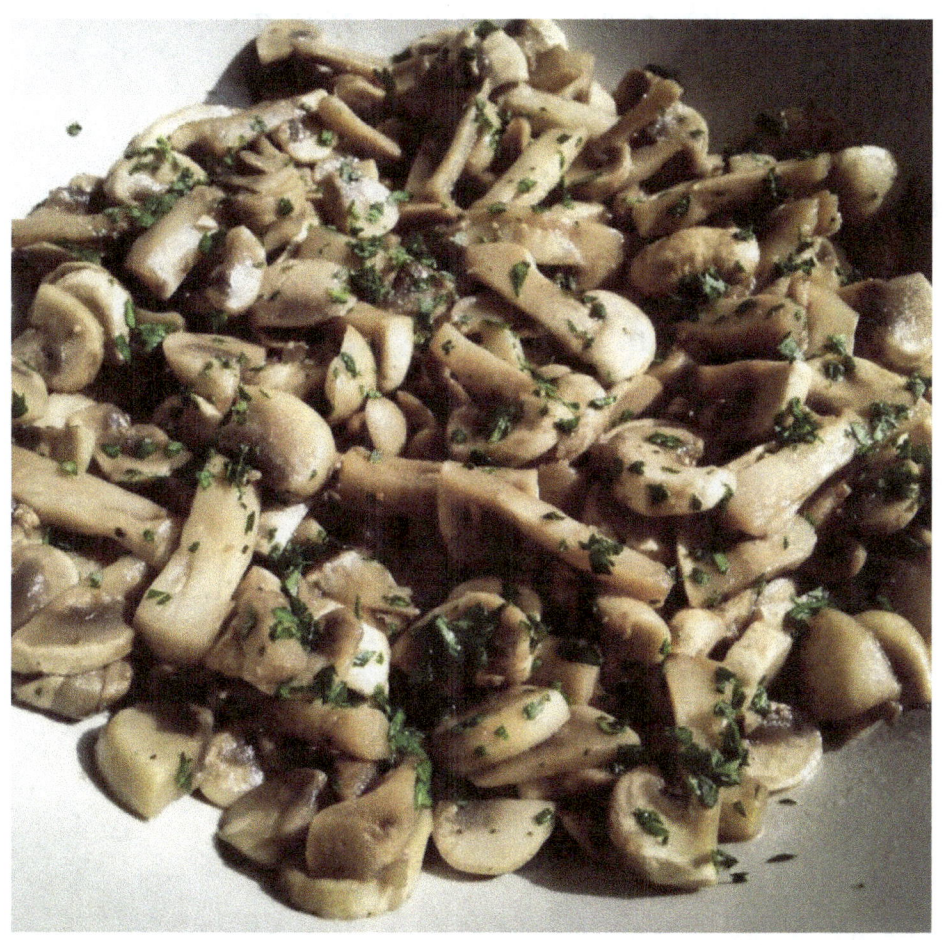

Corn Salad

Ingredients: 2 servings

- Cooked (or canned) corn, 100 gr.
- Bell pepper, ½
- Celery, 1/2 stalk
- Onion, ½
- Chili, ½
- Garlic, 1 clove
- Parsley, 1 sprig
- Juice of half a lemon
- Salt and pepper, to taste

Directions:

1) Drain the corn, cut the garlic, onion, chili, parsley, celery and pepper mixing them in order. Season with lemon juice and salt. Leave to macerate in the refrigerator for an hour. Enjoy your meal!

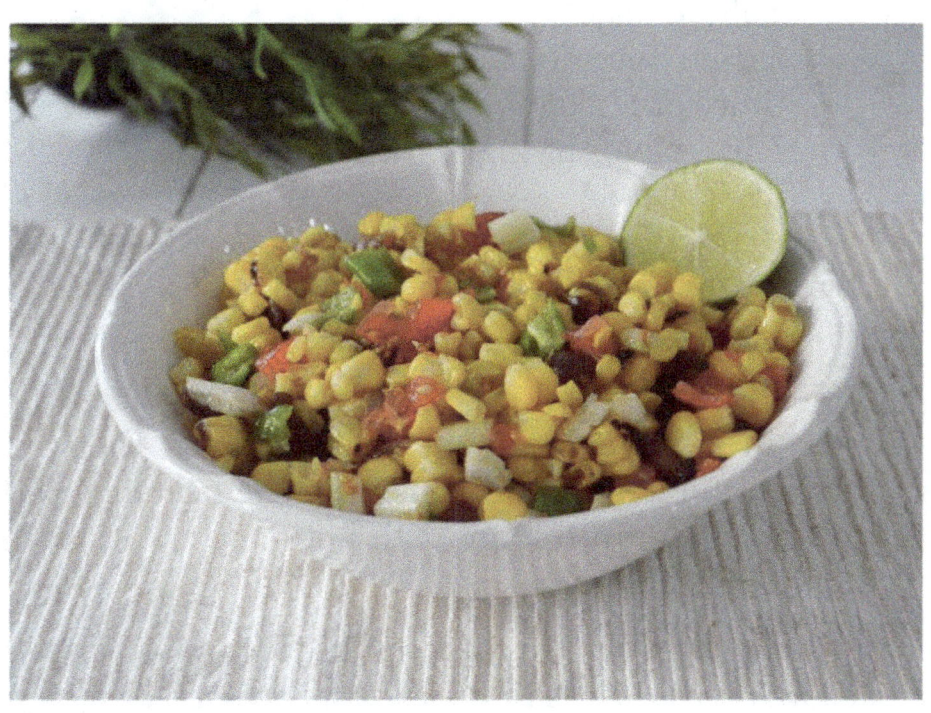

Breaded Artichokes

Ingredients: 2 servings

- 4 artichokes
- 1 egg
- Salt, to taste
- White flour, to taste
- Juice of 1/2 lemon
- Olive oil for frying, to taste

Directions:

1) Clean the artichokes by removing the hard leaves and fluff. Slice them into small pieces and immediately place them in water and lemon. Drain and dry them. Pass them in the flour and dip them in the beaten egg with salt. Dip them in the pot with hot oil. Fry. Stir so that each part is browned.

2) Remove and place them on kitchen paper sheets to absorb excess oil. Season with salt and serve. Enjoy your meal!

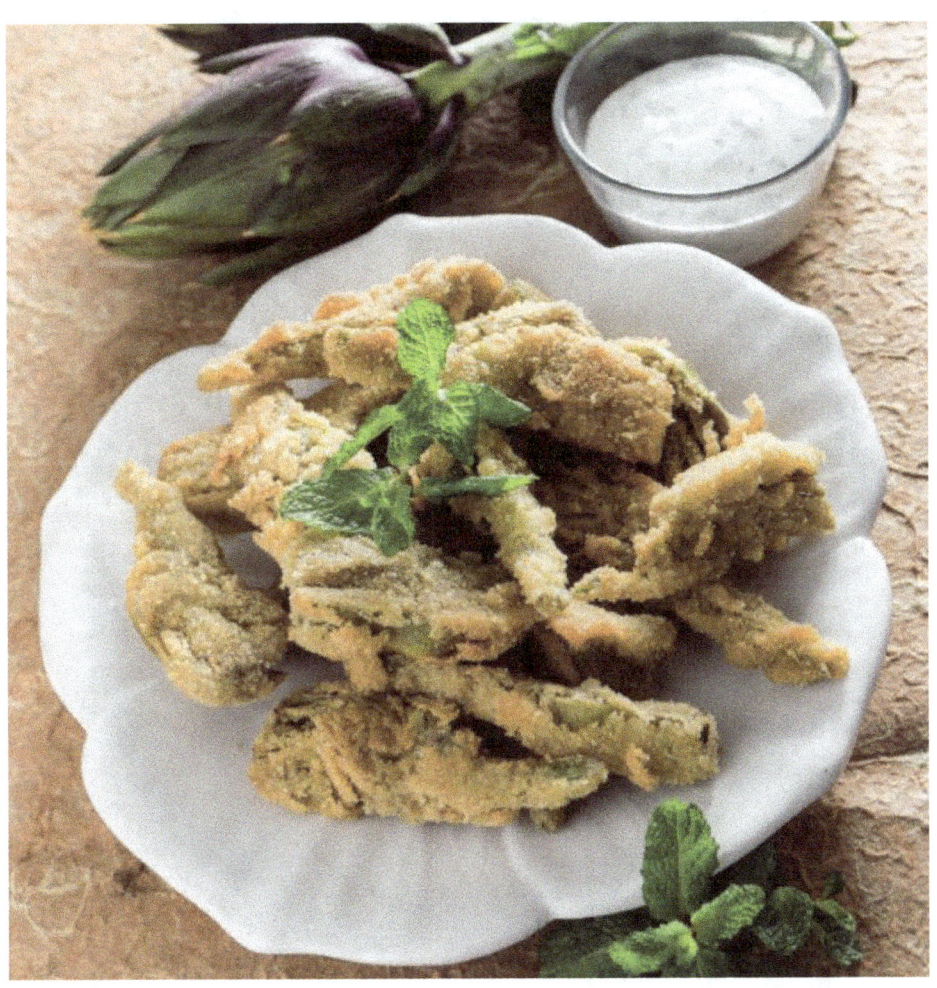

Sauteed Broccoli

Ingredients: 2 servings

- Broccoli, 340 gr.
- Extra virgin olive oil, to taste
- Garlic, 1/2 clove
- Chili pepper, a pinch
- Salt, to taste

Directions:

1) Rinse the broccoli. Chop them up. Boil them for 5 min. in salt water. Drain them. Put them in a pan with a drizzle of oil. Season with salt and a pinch of chili pepper. Serve hot. Enjoy your meal!

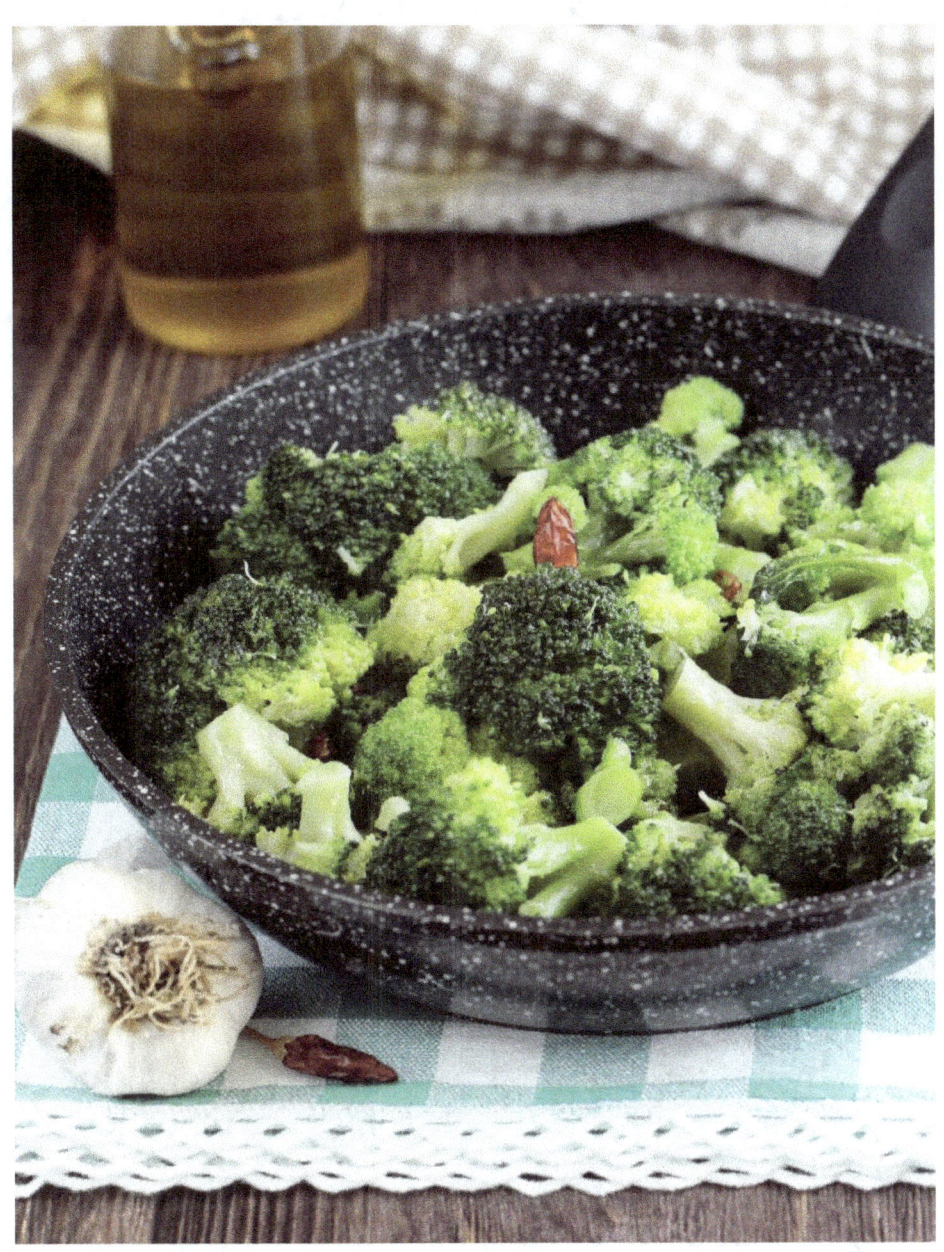

Sweet and Treats

Italian Babà

Ingredients: 1 babà

- Flour 0, 250 gr.
- Butter, 80 gr.
- Sugar, 25 gr.
- Yeast, 20 gr.
- 5 eggs
- Salt, a pinch
- Water, 1 dl.
- Sugar, 100 gr.
- Rum, 1 small glass

Directions:

1) Dissolve the yeast in a little warm water. Knead a dough with 50 gr. of flour. Let it rise until it is well swollen.

2) Put the leavened dough in a bowl. Combine the rest of the flour, salt and eggs. Work everything very vigorously until the dough comes off the sides of the bowl.

3) Add the sugar and melted butter mixing well. Put the dough in a babà shape with very high edges (after having floured and buttered it) and let it rise until the dough has doubled its volume.

4) Bake for 40 minutes in a preheated oven at 180°C.Finish cooking when the surface of the babà has a nice burnished color. Let the cake cool. Then wet it with the syrup obtained by dissolving the water and sugar on the stove. Once cooled add the rum. Enjoy your meal!

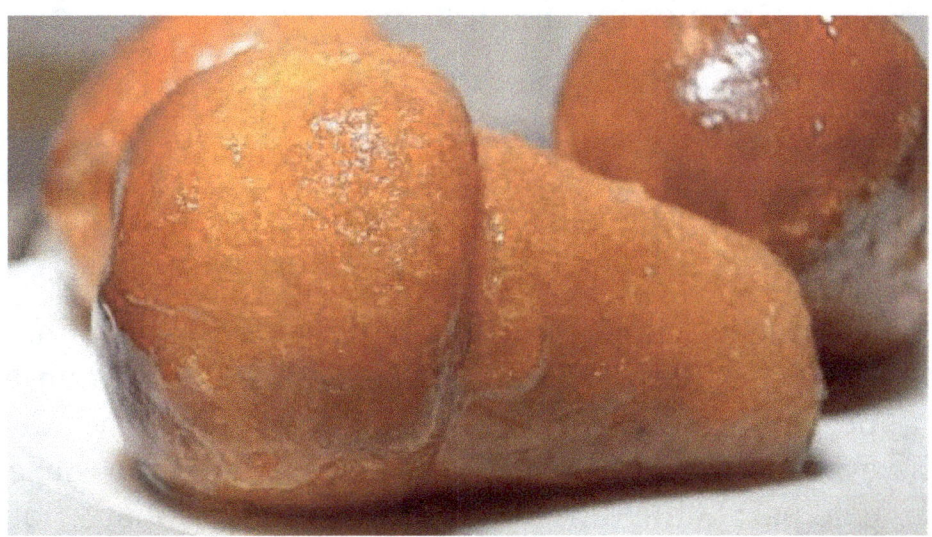

Cinnamon Cookies

Ingredients: 2 servings

- White flour, 100 gr.
- Softened butter, 80 gr.
- Powdered sugar, 40 gr. (to taste and to garnish)
- 2 hard-boiled egg yolks
- Grated peel of 1/2 lemon
- Ground cinnamon, 1 tsp

Directions:

1) Sieve the egg yolks. Pass the flour through a sieve as well. Place it like a fountain on a work base.

2) Place the chopped butter in the center of the fountain. Combine the powdered sugar. Add the cinnamon and pureed egg yolks. Work the dough quickly. Cover everything with cling paper. Place the dough in the least cold part of the refrigerator. Let it rest for about 3 hours.

3) Resume the dough after the time has elapsed. Roll it out with a rolling pin giving it a height of 3 mm. Use a pastry cutter or mold and shape the cookies. Arrange them in a previously greased and floured plate. Move them to a preheated oven at 180°C. For about 15 min. Check the cooking. Remove and let cool. Sprinkle with powdered sugar. Serve. Enjoy your meal!

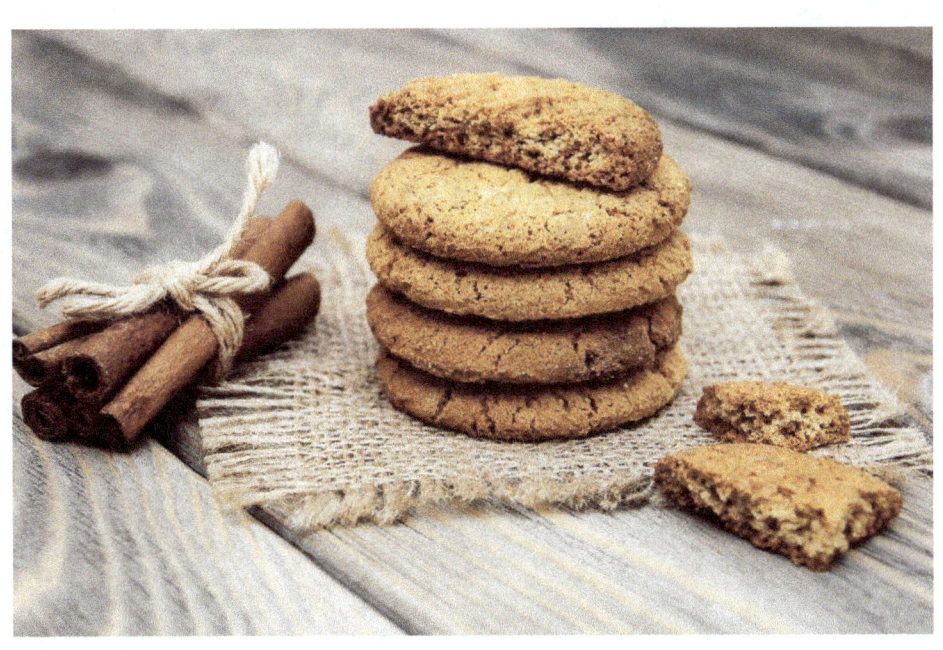

Eggnog

Ingredients: 2 servings

- Granulated sugar, 40 gr.
- Dry marsala, 40 gr.
- 2 eggs

Directions:

1) Whip the egg yolks in a bowl. Dilute with the poured Marsala and continue to work the mixture. Cook in a bain-marie with low flame. Continue whipping until you have a soft cream. Remove when the cream has a good consistency. Enjoy your meal!

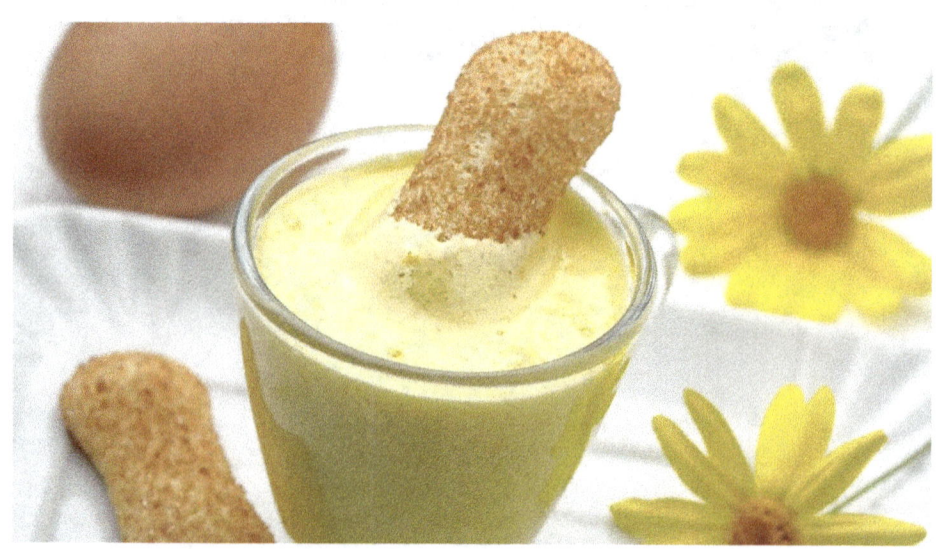

Hazelnut Ice Cream

Ingredients: 2 servings

- hazelnuts, 100 gr.
- Sugar, 170 gr.
- Milk, 750 cl.
- Vanilla sugar, 1 sachet
- 6 egg yolks

Directions:

1) Remove the skin from the hazelnuts. To do this you have to blanch them in boiling water (not too much, they must not cook). Put them in the blender. Reduce them to a pulp. Add 2 tablespoons of milk to the hazelnuts.

2) Pour the rest of the milk into a saucepan. Boil it together with the vanilla sugar. Pour everything into the hazelnuts. Mix well. Let the mixture rest for half an hour.

3) Work the egg yolks with the sugar. Slowly combine the hazelnut mixture. Cook everything over low heat, always continuing to stir. Be careful it doesn't stick. Remove from the heat as soon as the cream begins to boil. Let it cool and then put it in the ice cream maker for about 20 minutes. Enjoy your meal!

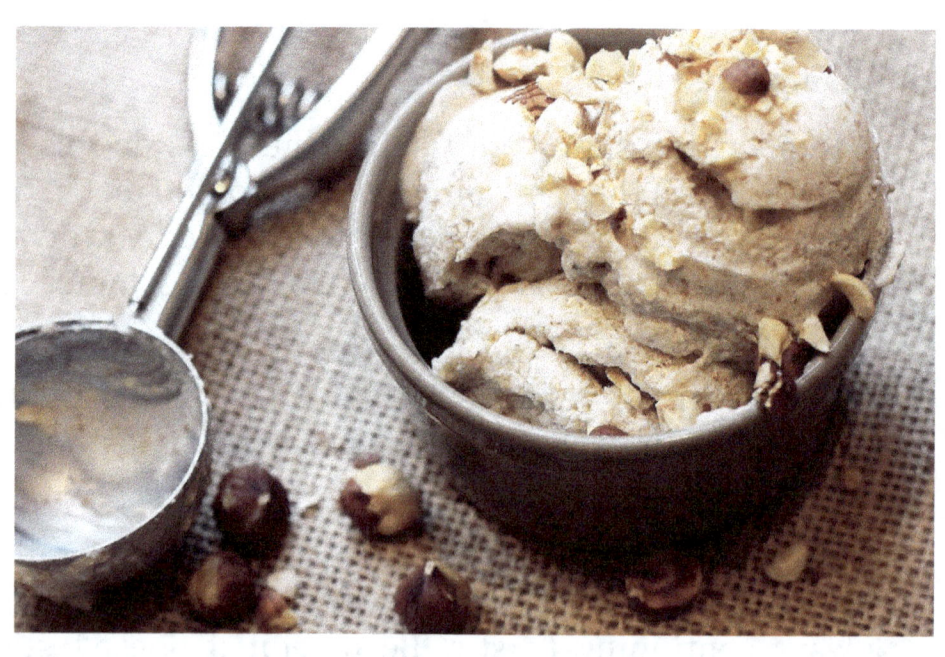

Profiteroles

Ingredients: 2 servings

For the bignè pastry:

- water, 1/4 l.
- Butter, 125 gr.
- Salt, 1 pinch
- White flour, 150 gr.
- 2 whole eggs

Other ingredients:

- Whipped cream, 200 gr.
- Powdered sugar, a few tablespoons
- Chocolate sauce, 4 dl.

Directions:

1) In a saucepan that is not too large, bring the water to a boil with the margarine and salt. Remove the saucepan from the heat and pour in the flour, stirring constantly.

2) Put the mixture back on the heat and let it cook for another 5 minutes, until the dough detaches from the walls. Pour it into a bowl and let it cool. Then add the whole eggs one at a time, beating vigorously.

3) Keep whisking until the dough forms bubbles. Put it in a syringe with a smooth metal mouth.

By pressing, bring out on the greased oven plate some balls as big as a walnut, keeping them 4 cm away from each other. Cook them in a moderate oven (180°C) without opening it during cooking for about 20 minutes.

When cooked, the inside of the bignè must be completely empty and dry.

4) Remove them from the oven and let them cool on a wire rack. Open them on one side with scissors and fill them with the lightly sweetened whipped cream. Arrange them in a dome shape on the plate and pour the chocolate sauce over them. Enjoy your meal!

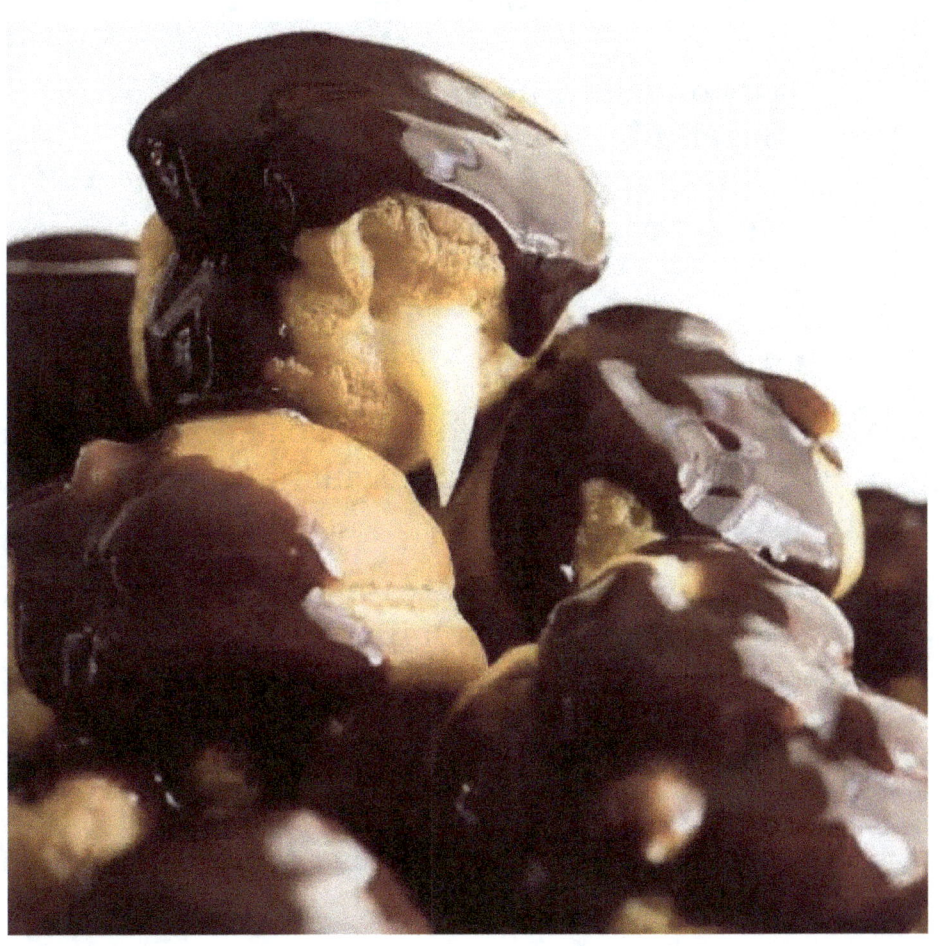

Sweet Salami

Ingredients: 2 servings

- 1 egg
- Sweet cocoa powder, 1 hg.
- Butter, 1 hg.
- Dry biscuits, 1 hg.
- Sugar, 1 hg.
- Sambuca (or other sweet liqueur), 1/2 glass
- 1 sheet of greaseproof paper

Directions:

1) Put the egg, sugar, butter in a baking dish and mix well. Add cocoa, chopped biscuits and liqueur to the mixture.

2) Pour everything on the greaseproof paper and roll up. Tie like salami and place in the freezer for a couple of days. Serve cold and cut into slices. Enjoy your meal!

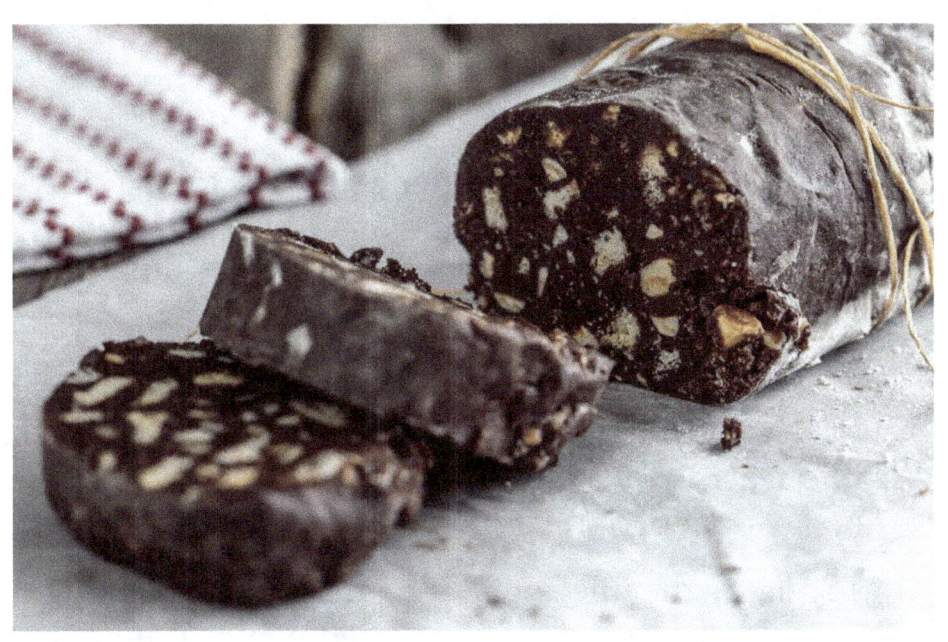

Lemon Sorbet

Ingredients: 2 servings

- 7 lemons
- Egg white, ½
- Sugar, 100 gr.

Directions:

1) Wash and dry 1 lemon, cut the zest taking only the yellow part (because the white inside is very bitter), then with a very sharp knife cut it into very thin and short filaments.

2) Wash and dry 2 other large lemons with the peel intact, cut them in half, then empty the pulp with a small knife leaving only the thickness of the peel. Dry them and keep them in the refrigerator.

3) Squeeze the juice of all the other lemons, taking care to reach 10 cl in total, if you need you can increase the number of lemons. Melt the sugar over low heat in 180 cl. of water, and when diluted let it cool, add the filaments of zest, lemon juice and leave to infuse for 1 hour.

4) Whip the egg white that you have kept at room temperature until stiff and add it to the mixture. Fill all the half lemons and place them in the freezer, where they should be kept for up to 10 minutes before serving. Enjoy your meal!

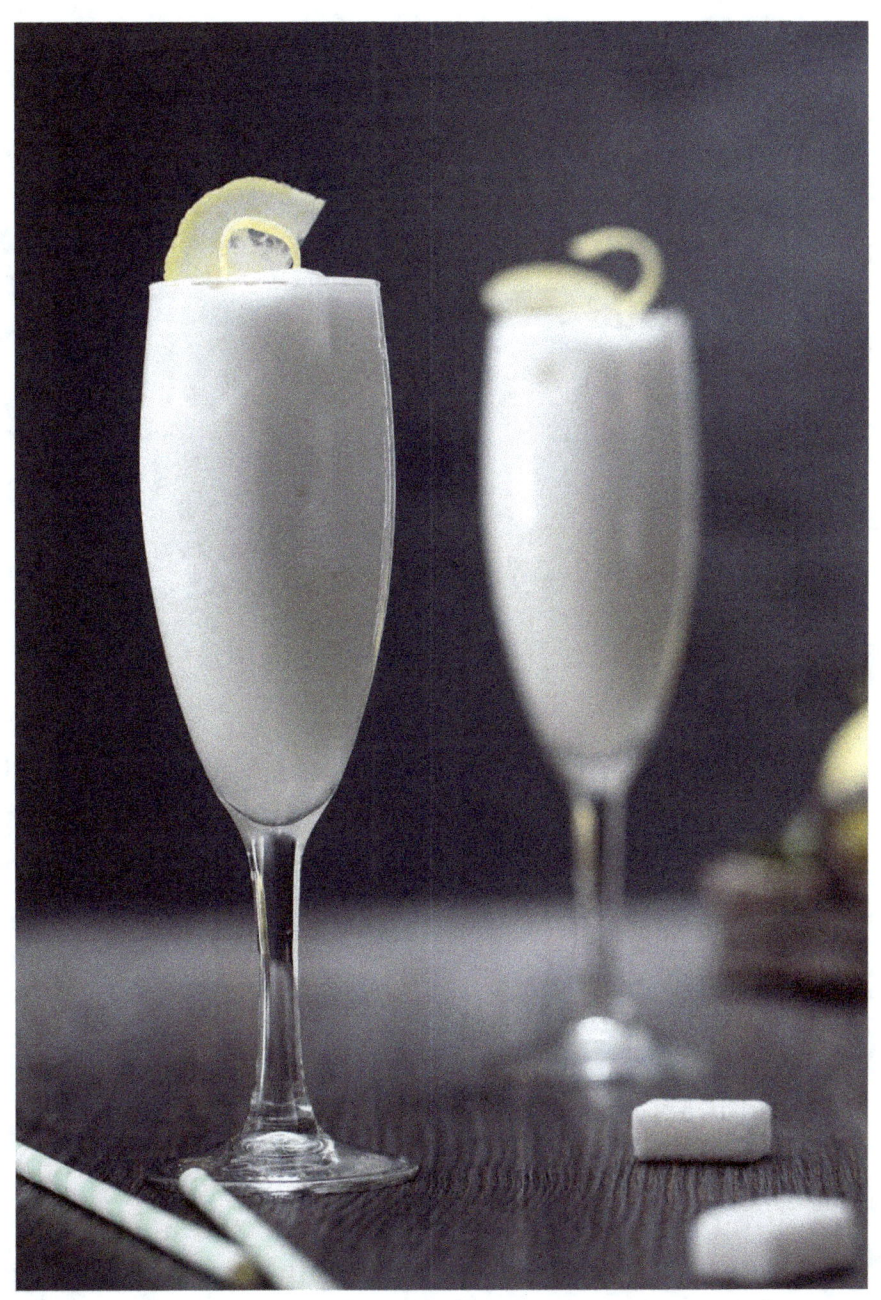

Cannoncini with Cream

Ingredients: 2 servings

- Frozen puff pastry, 1 pack
- Powdered sugar, 50 gr.
- 1 egg

For the custard:

- 2 egg yolks
- Sugar, 25 gr.
- Flour, 25 gr.
- Milk, 1/4 l.
- Vanilla sugar, 1 sachet

Directions:

1) Defrost the puff pastry in time. Make the custard. With a wooden spoon, whisk the egg yolks with the sugar. Gradually add the sifted flour and hot milk. Scent with vanilla or lemon zest.

2) Bring the cream to a boil over medium heat and let it boil for 5 minutes, stirring constantly. Let it cool, stirring it from time to time or veiling it with a little melted margarine to avoid the skin on the surface.

3) Roll out the puff pastry, a few millimeters thick, with a rolling pin. Cut it into strips 1 cm wide and about 15 cm long. Wrap each strip in a spiral around the special metal torch greased with margarine, slightly

overlapping the dough. Press the dough from one end to close two cannoli.

4) Brush the cannoncini with beaten egg. Line them up on the greased oven plate. Sprinkle them with powdered sugar and bake them in a hot oven (200°C) for about 10 minutes. Remove them from the oven and let them cool. Gently remove them from the torches and, with the help of a pastry syringe or a teaspoon, fill them with the prepared cream. Enjoy your meal!

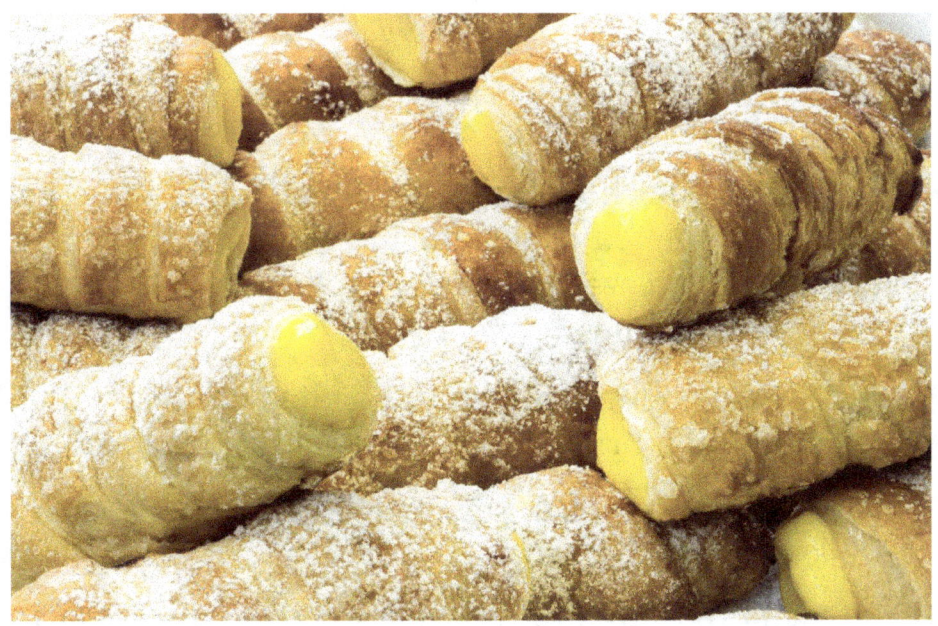

Coffee Chocolates

Ingredients: 2 servings

- Dark chocolate, 200 gr.
- 3 egg yolks
- Sugar, 80 gr.
- Milk, 250 ml.
- 1 tablespoon of flour
- 1 sachet of vanillin
- 2 tablespoons of instant coffee
- 30 coffee beans
- Paper cups, to taste

Directions:

1) Temper the chocolate. Brush the inside of the paper cups with melted chocolate and let it solidify (you can also let the freezer help you ...!). Repeat the operation for at least 4 times.

2) Dip the coffee beans in the melted chocolate and let them solidify. Bring milk and instant coffee to a boil.

3) Beat the egg yolks, sugar, flour and vanilla. Add the milk and mix.

4) Bring the mixture to a boil for 8 minutes and let it cool. Remove the chocolate from the cups and pour in the coffee cream. Decorate the chocolates with chocolate-covered coffee beans. Enjoy your meal!

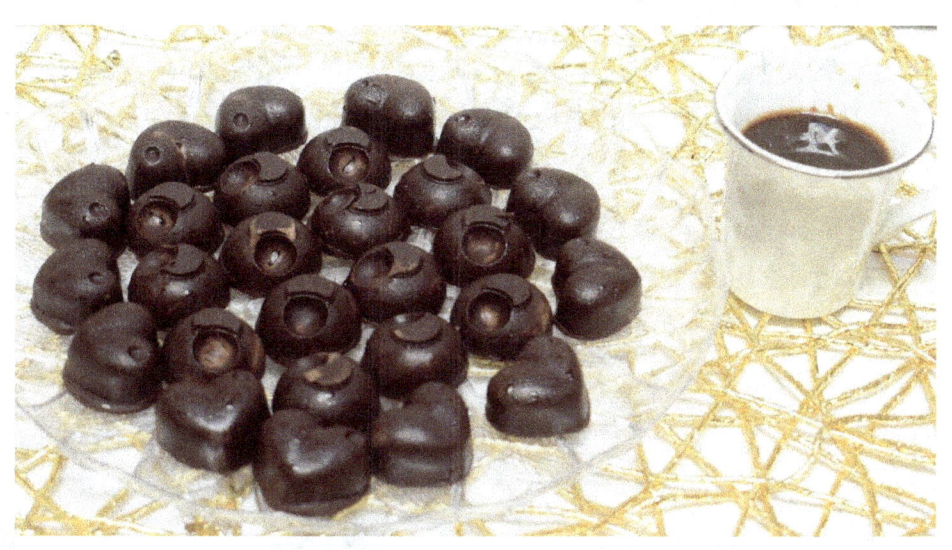

Blueberry Jam

Ingredients: 2 servings

- Blueberry
- Sugar

Directions:

1) Wash the blueberries and mix them cold with the same amount of sugar. Let them macerate for a few hours.

2) Cook everything for about 15 minutes, skimming often. Place the jam in the jars. Let it cool down. Close tightly and keep cool. Enjoy your meal!

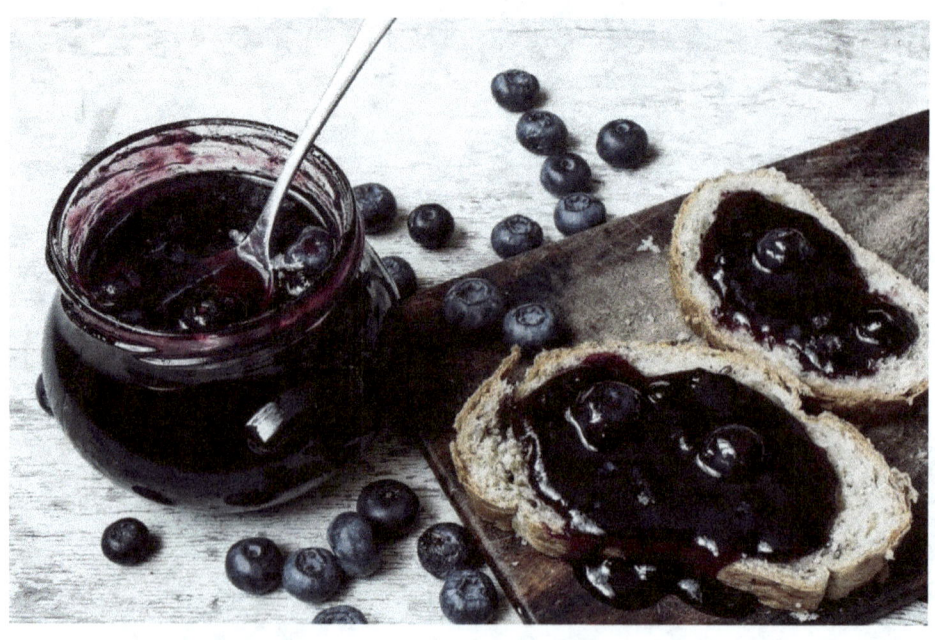

www.ingramcontent.com/pod-product-compliance
Lightning Source LLC
Chambersburg PA
CBHW071529080526
44588CB00011B/1616